BACK PAIN IN THE WORKPLACE

Mission Statement of IASP Press

The International Association for the Study of Pain (IASP) is a nonprofit, interdisciplinary organization devoted to understanding the mechanisms of pain and improving the care of patients with pain through research, education, and communication. The organization includes scientists and health care professionals dedicated to these goals. The IASP sponsors scientific meetings and publishes newsletters, technical bulletins, the journal *Pain*, and books.

The goal of IASP Press is to provide the IASP membership with timely, high-quality, attractive, low-cost publications relevant to the problem of pain. These publications are also intended to appeal to a wider audience of scientists and clinicians interested in the problem of pain.

We will achieve high-quality publications through careful selection of subjects and authors, well-focused editorial work at several levels of production, and a smooth flow of materials. In addition, we believe that we can restrain costs and prices by employing the administrative resources of the IASP central office and by obtaining grant support for selected publications.

Because we will keep the price of our books low and their value high, they will reach a wider audience than do similar books published by for-profit companies. Furthermore, our access to leaders in the field of pain research and treatment guarantees an outstanding selection of material and excellent editorial oversight.

Recent publications from IASP Press

Visceral Pain, edited by Gerald F. Gebhart

Temporomandibular Disorders and Related Pain Conditions, edited by Barry J. Sessle, Patricia S. Bryant, and Raymond A. Dionne

Touch, Temperature, and Pain in Health and Disease: Mechanisms and Assessments, edited by Jörgen Boivie, Per Hansson, and Ulf Lindblom

Classification of Chronic Pain: Descriptions of Chronic Pain Syndromes and Definitions of Pain Terms, Second Edition, Task Force on Taxonomy, edited by H. Merskey and N. Bogduk

Proceedings of the 7th World Congress on Pain, edited by Gerald F. Gebhart, Donna L. Hammond, and Troels S. Jensen

Pharmacological Approaches to the Treatment of Chronic Pain: New Concepts and Critical Issues, edited by Howard L. Fields and John C. Liebeskind

BACK PAIN IN THE WORKPLACE

MANAGEMENT OF DISABILITY IN
NONSPECIFIC CONDITIONS

a report of the

Task Force on Pain in the Workplace
of the
International Association for the Study of Pain

Chairman and Editor

Wilbert E. Fordyce, PhD
Department of Rehabilitation Medicine
University of Washington
Seattle, Washington, USA

IASP PRESS • SEATTLE

Library of Congress Cataloging-in-Publication Data

Back pain in the workplace : management of disability in nonspecific conditions :
    a report of the Task Force on Pain in the Workplace of the International
    Association for the Study of Pain / chairman and editor, Wilbert E. Fordyce.
        p.   cm.
    Includes bibliographical references and index.
    ISBN 0-931092-11-6 (paperbound)
    1. Backache. 2. Occupational diseases. 3. Disability evaluation. I. Fordyce,
Wilbert E.   II. International Association for the Study of Pain. Task Force on
Pain in the Workplace.
    [DNLM: 1. Low Back Pain—prevention & control. 2. Occupational
Diseases. 3. Disability Evaluation.   WE 755 P144 1995]
RD771.B217P35 1995
617.5'64—dc20
DNLM/DLC
for Library of Congress   95-16905

IASP Press
International Association for the Study of Pain
909 NE 43rd St., Suite 306
Seattle, WA 98105 USA
Fax: 206-547-1703

Printed in the United States of America

Contents

Members* and Consultants** of the Task Force on Pain in the Workplace

Richard E. Atkinson, MB BS* *Pain Management Clinic, Chesterfield and North Derbyshire Royal Hospital, Chesterfield, Derbyshire, UK*

Michelle Battié, RPT, ScD** *Department of Orthopaedics, University of Washington, Seattle, Washington, USA*

Richard J. Butler, PhD** *Industrial Relations Center, University of Minnesota, Minneapolis, Minnesota, USA*

Eric J. Cassell, MD** *Professor of Public Health, Cornell University Medical College, New York, NewYork, USA*

Richard Deyo, MD** *Health Services Research and Development, University of Washington, Seattle, Washington, USA*

Wilbert E. Fordyce, PhD* *Department of Rehabilitation Medicine, University of Washington, Seattle, Washington, USA*

Gary M. Franklin, MD** *Department of Labor and Industries, Olympia, Washington, USA*

Rochelle Habeck, PhD** *Department of Educational Psychology and Special Education, Michigan State University, East Lansing, Michigan, USA*

Larry Kenney** *Washington State Labor Council (AFL-CIO), Seattle, Washington, USA*

Masaharu Kumashiro, PhD** *Department of Ergonomics, Institute of Industrial Ecological Sciences, University of Occupational and Environmental Health, Kitakyushu, Japan*

John D. Loeser, MD* *Departments of Neurological Surgery and Anesthesiology and Multidisciplinary Pain Center, University of Washington, Seattle, Washington, USA*

George Mendelson, MB BS, MD* *Pain Management Centre, Caulfield General Medical Centre, Caulfield, Victoria, Australia*

Alf Nachemson, MD* *Department of Orthopaedic Surgery, Sahlgren Hospital, Goteborg, Sweden*

Margareta Nordin, RPT, PhD** *Occupational and Industrial Orthopaedic Center, Hospital for Joint Diseases Orthopaedic Institute, New York, New York, USA*

Marian Osterweis, PhD** *Association of Academic Health Centers, Washington, District of Columbia, USA*

Patricia M. Owens, MPA** *Disability Programs, UNUM Life Insurance Company of America, New York, New York, USA*

Issy Pilowsky, MD* *Department of Psychiatry, The University of Adelaide, Royal Adelaide Hospital, Adelaide, South Australia, Australia*

Joel Seres, MD* *Northwest Pain Center, Portland, Oregon, USA*

Erik Spangfort, MD, PhD* *Department of Orthopaedic Surgery, Huddinge University Hospital, Huddinge, Sweden*

Walter C. Stolov, MD** *Department of Rehabilitation Medicine, University of Washington, Seattle, Washington, USA*

Alan H. Strohmeier, LLB** *Unemployment and Workers Compensation, General Motors Corporation, Detroit, Michigan, USA*

Ronald B. Tasker, MD* *Toronto Western Hospital, Toronto, Ontario, Canada*

Ernest Volinn, PhD* *Multidisciplinary Pain Center, University of Washington, Seattle, Washington, USA*

Gordon Waddell, DSc, MD* *Orthopaedic Department, Western Infirmary, Glasgow, UK*

Edward Yelin, PhD** *Department of Medicine and Health Policy, University of California, San Francisco, San Francisco, California, USA*

Foreword

In that substantial segment of the population referred to as the working age group, low back pain is the most prevalent "medical" condition, the most costly, and the greatest cause of lost work days. The broad field of chronic pain includes many problems that are directly or indirectly related to the workplace. It is estimated that the health care costs of chronic pain exceed the combined costs of coronary artery disease, cancer, and AIDS. On that basis alone, pain in the workplace would seem an important medical, economic, and societal problem that is aptly described as a "hidden epidemic." However, as clearly outlined in this document, it would be inappropriate to regard pain in the workplace strictly as a medical problem with financial and societal consequences. As is the case for all chronic pain problems, physical, psychological, and environmental factors are interwoven. This is particularly so in the setting of the workplace.

The International Association for the Study of Pain (IASP) was established to foster interaction among health professionals from a broad range of disciplines and basic scientists with a common interest in research and treatment of all forms of pain. The IASP also encourages participation from individuals outside of the health care professions whose interest or expertise impinge on some aspect of pain research or treatment. Thus the IASP was an ideal organization to bring together a diverse range of individuals and draw upon this combined expertise, to provide a clear description of the complex issues involved, and to suggest strategies for prevention and treatment of pain in the workplace. Such advice is urgently needed to address the rapidly escalating costs in terms of human suffering, lost productivity, and a massive financial burden.

I am pleased that the work of the Task Force on Pain in the Workplace, which has resulted in this publication, was begun during my term as president of IASP. My immediate choice to head this task force was Professor Wilbert E. Fordyce, who had clearly played a key role in this field, drawing our attention to environmental influences on pain behavior and establishing the use of cognitive/behavioral methods for treatment of chronic pain, as well as emphasizing important strategies for prevention of chronicity. Professor Fordyce assembled a task force of extraordinary diversity and persevered with the extremely difficult tasks of collating an enormous range of information and obtaining consensus in the majority of cases. This publication represents the distillation of the highly specialized input of persons from many disciplines from throughout the world. I have no doubt that it will represent a landmark, enhancing knowledge concerning pain in the workplace and setting a logical framework for important advances in prevention and treatment.

MICHAEL J. COUSINS, MD
Professor and Director
Pain Management and Research Centre
University of Sydney
Royal North Shore Hospital
Sydney, Australia

Preface

In furtherance of its educational mission, the International Association for the Study of Pain (IASP) set up a Task Force on Pain in the Workplace (PIW) to study and report recommendations for the management of disability in nonspecific low back pain (NSLBP). The project arose because of clear evidence that rates of disability assignment and duration of disability status from NSLBP have been increasing rapidly in economically developed countries. These increases pose threats to the personal and economic well-being of injured workers and their families, and to the economic viability of employers and industry, of health insurance and compensation agencies, and of taxpayers.

This document grew out of the interest of the IASP Council to reach beyond health care delivery into the broader community of the countries represented in this international organization to share knowledge and recommend new management procedures for NSLBP, a common health care, wage replacement, and administrative issue. The task force was constituted in 1989, under the direction of then IASP President Dr. Michael Cousins. Its work has continued under the presidencies of Dr. Ulf Lindblom and Dr. John Loeser.

To create this report, the task force divided the broad topical area into six domains. Members and consultants of PIW were asked to write mini-papers setting forth synopses of their individual views and the information available about a given domain. Each member then wrote two or three review papers, ensuring breadth of coverage and multiple viewpoints. These mini-papers were collated and circulated to all members and consultants.

Through the generosity of the Volvo Research Foundation, funding was obtained for a two-day meeting of many of the members and consultants. Mini-papers and selected supporting documents were provided to attendees prior to the meeting. At the meeting, which was held in Seattle, Washington, on October 11–12, 1992, proposed recommendations were formulated.

The chairman of this task force subsequently undertook the task of collating and integrating the recommendations, reviewing the nature and scope of the problem, and reviewing the pertinent literature. The writing process was marked by frequent communications and exchanges between the chairman and various members of PIW. Further, a meeting of several PIW members occurred at the 7th World Congress on Pain in Paris, France, in August 1993. A preliminary presentation of PIW proposals was made at that meeting and at the November 1993 meeting of the American Pain Society in Orlando, Florida, USA. Those presentations provided for discussion periods and permitted further feedback from interested persons outside the Task Force.

A draft of the PIW report was circulated to all members and consultants, and their critiques and suggestions were assimilated into a redraft that was reviewed by three referees familiar with the topic but unfamiliar with the report. It is impossible to pinpoint which ideas or proposals came from which person or persons, except as may be explicitly stated in the text. Members and consultants did not all speak with one voice. Accordingly, each member or consultant may disagree with parts of the PIW report. The final report reflects the chairman's judgments as to what best to say to capture the consensus and provide a coherent and integrated document.

IASP and the Task Force on Pain in the Workplace thank the Volvo Research Foundation for its financial support of the task force meeting. Other support for this project was provided by IASP.

WILBERT E. FORDYCE, PHD

Executive Summary

This book contains the recommendations of the Task Force on Pain in the Workplace of the International Association for the Study of Pain. It concerns prevention of back pain disability. It deals with worksite-based interventions to minimize disability, a program to substitute job-change flexibility for inappropriate disability assignment, early medical management of disability for nonspecific low back pain (NSLBP), and early and long-term disability management when early medical management fails to lead to return to work. Recommendations were formulated with due regard for the welfare of injured workers and their families, employers, health insurance and compensation agencies, and society as a whole. Potential legal issues were also considered.

Chronic NSLBP was conceptualized from the perspective of a biopsychosocial model. Within that framework, the principal features of policy recommendations are:

1. To reconceptualize NSLBP as a problem of *activity* intolerance, not a medical problem, in line with the United States Agency for Health Care Policy Research (AHCPR) Guidelines (Bigos 1994a) and the United Kingdom Clinical Standards Advisory Group Report (CSAG 1994).

2. To emphasize worksite-based interventions as a method for minimizing and limiting disability.

3. To structure medical management of NSLBP on a time-contingent rather than a pain-contingent basis.

4. To provide comprehensive reevaluation in cases where function is not restored and return to work is not achieved, including social and vocational assessment components.

5. To limit permanent disability status to conditions where irremediable impairment exists.

6. To define temporary disability as not requiring irremediable impairment.

7. To avoid consideration of psychological/psychiatric conditions attributed to pain for disability assignment as pain.

8. To reclassify as unemployed those who fail to achieve restoration of function and return to work, in line with reconceptualizing NSLBP as activity intolerance.

9. To establish vocational redirection programs for the unemployed.

10. To reanalyze disability policies bearing on all nonspecific and psychiatric/psychologic conditions.

With the concurrence of appropriate agencies, guideline recommendations for medical management of low back pain prepared for the United States by the AHCPR and for the United Kingdom by the CSAG have been summarized and inserted into this report (Chapter 7).

Back Pain in the Workplace: Management of Disability in Nonspecific Conditions, edited by W.E. Fordyce, IASP Press, Seattle, © 1995.

1

Introduction

Disability benefits are a form of support intended to protect the economic well-being of injured workers until they regain function and can resume productive work. Disability programs pertaining to low back pain have shown rapidly increasing incidence of claims, duration of disability status, and cost. These increases are occurring without evidence that back injuries are becoming more frequent or more severe. Moreover, disability is awarded increasingly frequently for back pain occurring in the absence of evidence of *specific* back injury.

Disability benefit programs and the essential protection they provide to injured workers and their families are seriously threatened by escalating costs that undermine their future. Trends in costs of disability programs for low back pain are ominous. The number of persons assigned to disability status is growing at an alarming rate in many countries. In the United States low back pain disability is growing at a discernibly higher rate than the aggregate of all other categories of disability (Volinn et al. 1991), and similar patterns are noted in most economically developed countries.

Disability ascribed to low back pain has highly visible costs but also extensive hidden costs, particularly in human suffering and threat to survival of the family unit. Assignment to disability status for chronic low back pain is a threat to the health of the injured worker, for it may expose the worker to potentially debilitating circumstances such as prescription of excessive rest, well-intentioned but ultimately harmful treatments, or overprotection by zealous family members. Any of these may lead to diminished health and to increased suffering by patient and family. Employers incur losses from diminished economic productivity. Rapidly accelerating health care and disability compensation costs are already enormous. If current trends continue, disability and health care benefit funds could ultimately be bankrupted.

Disability attributed to pathoanatomical dysfunction due to a work-related injury is the cornerstone of existing disability programs. Such programs use an impairment-rating disability system. Illness or injury leading to restriction of the "whole person's" capacity to perform triggers consideration of disability assignment. Disability benefits may be awarded if a pathoanatomical defect is demonstrated or inferred.

Persisting disability existing for reasons in whole or in part not attributable to pathoanatomical defect is a different matter. The increasing frequency and duration of disability assignment in the absence of increased incidence of specific low back pain injuries suggest that an impairment-rating approach is flawed. This report examines these flaws and suggests alternatives. It seeks to clarify the nature of disability and of the forces that exert distorting effects on disability programs and proposes policy, procedural, and conceptual changes designed to correct the distorting effects.

Disability programs are at the cusp of the balance between the needs of the individual and those of society. Although consideration will be given to the needs of the individual, the major focus of this report is the ways in which society deals with disability attributed to nonspecific low back pain. In the end, if social and political mechanisms for dealing with disability are retooled to become more effective, there will remain the larger issue of how the needs of individuals unable to cope adequately with competitive employment can be met. We articulate some of the critical features and propose remedies for escalating disability costs.

TASK FORCE OBJECTIVES

The members and consultants of the Task Force on Pain in the Workplace believe that the proposals put forth in this document will improve the welfare of workers, employers, and society in general. We seek to diminish the risks to health that result when a worker is inappropriately designated as disabled. We encourage efficient, high-quality medical care and rehabilitation services. We believe that a significant subset of injured workers, who are suffering and are burdened with difficulties in coping with life and work demands, have problems that have been mis-identified as stemming from injury to the low back. They believe, as do many professionals working to help them, that a medical problem is responsible for their disability. The evidence suggests otherwise. Indeed, health care may play a major role in creating the disability. We seek to provide more accurate identification of the core problems of these workers and to focus upon them appropriately targeted interventions.

We seek opportunities to assist in modifying career goals, to avoid threats to family integrity, and to protect against the real threat to disability benefits posed by soaring medical and disability costs. We seek to retain and enhance the benefits to worker and employer alike of the economic productivity derived from healthy and valued workers.

For society, we seek to diminish incidence and duration of disability, with its attendant costs to employers and to agencies or programs providing medical and disability benefits. We also seek to diminish the risks inherent in excessive medical services and to diminish ambiguity in disability determination in non-specific low back pain (NSLBP)—ambiguity that often leads to litigation. Whenever litigation is involved, funds flow to attorneys and other legal costs and are diverted from the intended beneficiaries.

APPLICABILITY

The International Association for the Study of Pain is an international organization, and this report is intended for international use. However, countries have different governmental structures and policies pertaining to disability management of low back pain.

Precise applications of the guiding principles described in this book will vary according to the schemes for disability management in individual countries and even separate jurisdictions within a given country. The principles elaborated can be applied in any political or economic system that wishes to provide a "safety net" for those who are not gainfully employed.

Programs to reduce suffering for the worker and

costs for the employer or society will impact other social welfare and health programs. In some instances, costs and workload for other programs are likely to increase as our suggested changes are implemented. It is our intent, however, that proposed cost reductions in low back pain disability management not result in equivalent increases in other programs. If our recommendations are implemented appropriately, net reductions both in suffering and in global costs should result.

A report such as this cannot spell out all possible ripple-effect changes in other systems. We have attempted to identify obvious changes that other programs or systems need to consider. We have also tried to present a balanced account of the factors involved in disability matters pertaining to NSLBP so that the interests of the individual and of society are evenly assessed and met.

The task force recommendations are predicated upon an understanding of the concepts of pain and suffering, as well as the concepts of impairment and disability, for such understanding lies at the root of the problem. The reader also must consider the broader issue of the relation of disability programs to the societies in which they exist. Those tasks will be undertaken in later chapters.

Our focus in this book is on NSLBP relating to the world of work. Many of the principles and issues set forth are relevant to other conditions, for example, repetitive strain injury, occupational musculoskeletal disorders, job-related stress disorders, and cumulative trauma disorders, but it is beyond the scope of this report to consider those conditions except as they relate by analogy to NSLBP.

SCOPE OF ANALYSIS

This report clarifies the relationship of pain to suffering, impairment, and disability, and improves the focus on the problems facing suffering workers. The concepts and policies presented here suggest strategies for dealing with NSLBP, as well as disability problems above and beyond NSLBP.

Modification of NSLBP disability management must consider the problem from many different levels, as changes in one will influence others. The topography of the NSLBP problem includes medical or anatomical and physiological matters; it also includes workplace factors concerning ergonomic and accident or injury prevention programs and procedures for dealing with an injured worker who has reported back pain interfering with job performance. Another, even more important element is the growing awareness that the relationship of the worker to his or her job and employer plays a pivotal role in determining which workers seek health care intended to deal with their suffering.

Once a worker is involved with a health care provider, medical or health care management of the problem becomes a central concern, and is therefore a major focus of this report. The worker who has reported back pain and initiated medical care and promptly resumes normal work activity presents no significant problem with the management of back pain disability. Disability status becomes a problem if rapid return to work and resumption of normal activity do not occur. The condition of the employee is not the only factor influencing return to work. Barriers also come from the managing physician, employer, third-party insurance carriers, and compensation agencies.

A major part of the management problem concerns the definition of disability. This definition traditionally is based solely on complaints of pain and the processes by which it is judged to be present. Our review of disability determination procedures and our recommendations for change are found in Chapter 8.

Disability status also impacts family function, often adversely. Long-term management of the person on disability status is an important issue, involving medical management, employer policies regarding employment or reemployment of disabled workers, and compensation benefit management. The policies of each society concerning relationships of disability to medical benefits and to family maintenance support must also be considered. Societies usually have mechanisms for the injured worker to seek redress if existing medical treatment and disability management programs fail to restore employment. Attorneys may be retained by the injured worker to assist in protecting worker rights and benefits or to initiate legal action to seek to redress perceived failures of the system to provide expected benefits or protection. Those aspects of disability management also must be considered.

FOCUS: LOW BACK PAIN

This report provides a basis for a more rational way of dealing with the medical, social, and psychological factors that lead to long-term disability from NSLBP. The report does not present new data; it brings together existing knowledge to formulate solutions.

The problem of cost trends in disability management for low back pain pertains mainly to simple backache or NSLBP; that is, back pain complaints occurring without identifiable specific anatomical or neurophysiological causative factors. Nerve root problems and serious spinal pathology such as tumor, infection, and inflammatory disease, once identified, are quite distinct and separate (Waddell 1987). At the present state of medical knowledge, the following are known causes for specific back pain:

* Disk herniation.

* Spondylolisthesis, usually in the young.

* Spinal stenosis, usually in the elderly.

* Definite instability exceeding 4 to 5 mm on flexion/extension roentgenograms.

* Vertebral fractures, tumors, infections, and inflammatory diseases.

Patients with chronic true sciatica (i.e., pain in the low back and leg that radiates below the knee following a dermatomal distribution) probably belong in this list of causes. The best evidence suggests that fewer than 15% of persons with back pain can be assigned to one of these categories of specific low back pain (Spitzer et al. 1987). Medical science may find other specific causes for low back pain, but these are the ones we know today. Note that the conditions listed above are *not* the subject of this report.

Backache or NSLBP presents a particularly difficult example in the relationship of pain to suffering and disability. The complaint of pain and its relationship to suffering are ambiguous. The emotional processes underlying suffering are also unclear. Interactions between the person and his or her environment, both immediate and contextual, also contribute to the problem and make difficult the task of defining impairment and disability.

ENVIRONMENTAL AND CONTEXTUAL FACTORS

Traditionally, the individual is viewed as an independent entity functioning in an environment. That view, though having some validity, underestimates the extent to which human functioning is a product not only of characteristics or attributes of the individual but also of interactions of those with the environment. As Brown (1954) put it, "The new view holds that the human body is an organism which cannot be defined in terms of nonliving categories. . . . [This view] regards all disease as a total response to environmental threat. . . . [I]ts explanations are in social rather than biological terms."

The "unit" of concern in disability and NSLBP is not simply the person. The interactions between the person and the immediate environment blur the distinction between the two. Our concepts of pain, impairment, and disability must consider environmental factors as well as the person. Generally the most important aspects of environment are the workplace and the family.

Following a description of the nature and scope of the problem of disability management for NSLBP, this report reanalyzes the concepts of pain, impairment, and disability to provide a basis for recommended changes in how NSLBP disability is managed. The question should not be whether to change from our present systems, but what changes to make, and when. It should be understood, however, that change options implicate the basic values of a society. The nature and extent of the "contract" between an individual and the society, between the worker and the employer, and the obligations of each to the other, are fundamental to all that follows.

Back Pain in the Workplace: Management of Disability in Nonspecific Conditions, edited by W.E. Fordyce, IASP Press, Seattle, © 1995.

2

The Problem

INCIDENCE AND PREVALENCE TRENDS

Chronic pain complaints are common in economically developed countries. Bonica (1987) estimated that approximately 30% of the population of such countries suffer from chronic pain. Seventy million Americans report chronic pain, of whom more than 50 million are partially or totally disabled for periods ranging from a few days to weeks or months. Some are permanently disabled. A significant proportion of chronic pain problems relate to the low back.

Nachemson recently carried out an extensive review of the international literature on incidence of disabling low back pain (Nachemson 1992; Table 1). Disability from back pain clearly is a significant problem in each of the countries listed. Nachemson's report indicates that, great as the problem is in the

United States and Germany, it is even greater in Canada, Great Britain, The Netherlands, and Sweden.

Back pain is the second leading symptomatic reason for physician office visits in the United States (Lemrow et al. 1990). "Medical back problems" and "back and neck procedures age under 70" are the third and thirtieth most common reasons, respectively, for U.S. hospital admissions (Lemrow et al. 1990; Volinn 1991). The annual incidence rate of low back pain in the United States is estimated as 5% of the adult population (Frymoyer and Cats-Baril 1991), with a lifetime incidence or risk of 60–85% (Spengler et al. 1986; Von Korff and Dworkin 1989).

In a telephone survey of 1254 adult Americans, approximately 56% reported some back pain during the preceding year, with 3% reporting low back pain for more than 31 days (Sternbach 1986). Most of the

Table 1
Low back pain disability rates by country

Country	Population (millions)	Sick Days (millions per year)	Percentage of Work Force	Days Absent (per patient per year)	Level of Insurance Benefit (%)
United States [a,b,c]	240	20	2	9	0–80
Canada [d,e,f]	23	10	2	20	40–90
Great Britain [g,h]	55	33	2	30	0–80
West Germany [i,j,k]	61	16	4	10	100 (0–4 wks)* 80 (5–8 wks)* 60 (9 wks)*
The Netherlands [l,m]	14	4	4	25	80
Sweden					
1980 [n]	8	7	3	25	90
1983 [o]	8	13	5	30	90
1987 [p]	8.5	28	8	40	100

Sources: Adapted from Nachemson 1992. [a]Deyo and Tsui-wu 1987; [b]Frymoyer 1988; [c]Snook 1987; [d]Abenhaim and Suissa 1987; [e]Bombardier et al. 1985; [f]Lee et al. 1985; [g]Blow and Jayson 1988; [h]Wood and Bradley 1987; [i]Hettinger 1985; [j]Krämer 1989; [k]Kügelgen and Hillemacher 1985; [l]Valkenburg and Haanen 1982; [m]Zuidema 1985; [n]Chöler et al. 1985; [o]Riksförsäkringsverket 1987; [p]Nachemson 1991.
* Parentheses indicate duration of low back pain episode.

Table 2
Consequences of the back pain epidemic
in the United Kingdom

Sickness absence	52.6 million certified working days 1988–89 (largest single cause; 12.5% of total sick days)
Lost output	Estimated loss (1987–88) of £2 billion
General practitioner consults	Estimated 2 million annually
Hospital outpatient consults	Estimated 300,000 annually
Hospital inpatient episodes	Estimated 100,000 (1989–90)
Severe disability	50–1000 people severely affected in an average health district of 250,000 population

Source: Frank 1993.

respondents reported disability and health care utilization for their back pain. Frank (1993) reviewed the data on back pain in the United Kingdom. His findings are reported in Table 2. Further detail about the magnitude of the problem in the United Kingdom is reported by Walsh et al. (1992) and by Waddell (1994b); see Fig. 1.

Hager reported data on trends of industrial injury claims for back conditions during 1981–90 in the United States (1993; Fig. 2). These findings indicate that a high proportion of industrial injury claims relate to purported back injuries and that the proportion is increasing steadily. Similar trends are noted by Waddell (1994b) for back injury sick certification rates in the United Kingdom (Fig. 1). These data make clear that the award of disability for low back pain, already a major problem, is growing rapidly. This trend apparently is also true in other developing countries.

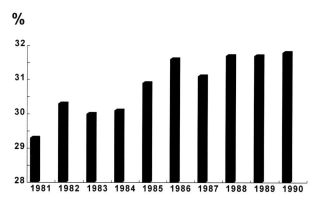

Fig. 2. Back claims as percentage of total claims in the United States. (Hager 1993. © 1993 NCCI. All rights reserved. Reprinted with permission.)

Award of disability status under the U.S. Social Security Disability Insurance (SSDI) program shows a comparable picture of rapid growth. During the 1970s the number of disabled workers receiving SSDI benefits doubled, the number of beneficiaries (disabled workers and their dependents) increased from 2.7 to 4.7 million, and cost of the program quintupled (Wiesmann and Deyo 1993). In the interval from SSDI program inception in 1957 through 1975, the average number of SSDI awards for the diagnostically questionable diagnosis of disk disease, using three-year averages, increased 2680% (Social Security Statistical Supplement 1979). Excellent summaries and review of the trend of increasing disability from low back pain and upper extremity pain can be found in Feuerstein (1993) and Hadler (1993).

Raspe (1993) reviewed the international literature on back pain, selecting four population studies as meeting adequate standards for data collection and analysis: Brattberg et al. 1989; Crook et al. 1984; Troup et al. 1987; and Von Korff and Dworkin 1989. These studies present data from Canada, Sweden, and the United States. The findings of the review were as follows (Raspe 1993):

1. Back pain is the first or second most prevalent pain complaint.

2. The average sufferer has a long history and multiple episodes. Chronic, continuous back pain accounts for maximally one quarter of the total prevalence.

3. The proportion of back pains that occur more than occasionally manifest themselves in a broad range of seriousness with 15% to 37% severe cases.

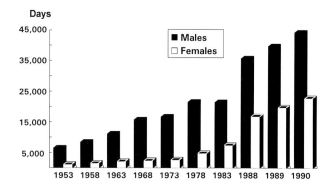

Fig. 1. Disability days per year in the United Kingdom. (Waddell 1994b)

4. Women are generally more often affected than men, though not statistically significantly so.

5. There is no unequivocal influence of age.

THE NATURAL COURSE OF BACK PAIN

Backache is common, as are brief intervals of restricted activity because of it, but most persons resume normal activities within a few days. Fewer than 20% of workers complaining of back pain they judged sufficiently severe to seek medical treatment continued to be off work at 40 days (Battié et al. 1993; Mayer et al. 1991). Back pain may occur as a single episode, continuous pain, or recurrent episodes of fluctuating severity. Each of those patterns has an unknown relationship to somatically based causative factors. The problem under consideration here is not the *incidence* of back pain. It is the *persistence,* following an incident, of pain complaints, health care consumption, and the inability to work, leading to disability status.

SPECIFIC VERSUS NONSPECIFIC BACK PAIN

Most back pain problems are nonspecific and self-limited in that no underlying pathophysiological or anatomical defects are found and they resolve within a few weeks (Andersson et al. 1983; Hadler 1993; Mayer et al. 1991; Philips and Grant 1991; Spengler et al. 1986). The crucial time is between 2 and 7–12 weeks, when pain that should be resolving fails to do so (Mayer et al. 1991; Spengler et al. 1986). Fig. 3 illustrates the typical time line of return to work for low back pain sufferers.

Back pain attributable to clearly identified patho-anatomic defect can be thought of as "specific" in that there is a specifiable source of nociceptive stimulation. Time to resolution of specific back pain problems is dictated by the particular pathoanatomic defect. Specificity of purported cause of back pain also has another connotation. Generalized degenerative processes accompanying aging or resulting from some disease process may lead to back pain. However, that is far from certain. The presence of degeneration does not in itself mean that there will be back pain. Everyone has some degree of "degeneration" with passage of time, but not everyone complains of back pain. Moreover, observation of complaints of back pain and

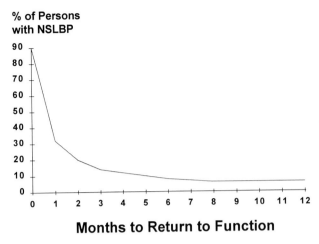

Fig. 3. Chronology of back pain: 80% of persons with nonspecific low back pain return to function in about two weeks, while fewer than 10% require five months or longer. (Mayer et al. 1991)

indications of degeneration does not establish a causal relationship. A common error in distinguishing between specific and nonspecific back pain is ascribing to injury what may be due to a chronic degenerative problem—an error that may be committed by the physician or the patient. Another frequent error is equating symptom flare with disease flare; again, by either physician or patient (Hadler 1992). Symptoms are influenced by events in the environment as well as by affective state (Pennebaker 1982). For many persons, suffering and complaints of back pain, as will be discussed in detail in Chapters 3, 4, and 5, are not reliably indicative of injury or a physiological or anatomical defect (Hadler 1992, 1994).

DISABILITY COSTS

Health care services and disability benefit costs correlate directly with award of disability status for back pain, though not necessarily with incidence or prevalence of the symptom. The magnitude of health care costs depends on the jurisdiction within which a given back pain case falls. Economic costs of disability from low back pain have effects throughout society. There is loss of economic productivity to the employer and to the overall economy. There is loss of tax revenue. Depending upon the availability and the monetary value of disability benefits, there almost certainly is economic loss for the worker and family. Disability and medical benefits draw from a pool of

Dollars per Employee

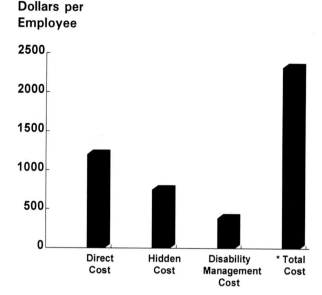

Fig. 4. Average cost of disability to 12 diverse businesses in the United States, showing direct and hidden costs of disability assignment and costs of disability management. * Total costs equal 8% of total payroll. (Modified from Chelius et al. 1992, © 1992 and published by Medical Economics at Montvale, NJ 07645; all rights reserved)

resources; therefore, each claim reduces the residual available for others who might need such assistance in the future.

Fig. 4 illustrates data on the impact of disability costs on businesses in the United States, showing cost distributions among direct and hidden effects of disability assignment and disability management procedures. In an article in the *New York Times* analyzing the impact of back pain disability on industry, the chief financial officer of a large American corporation said, "Workers' compensation . . . is a major American tragedy. People don't realize that the abuse of workers' comp is causing the loss of our own jobs" (Kerr 1993b).

Many variables influence the monetary costs of disability from low back pain. It is impractical to catalog these variables in different countries; however, a sampling of U.S. cost trends was recently prepared by the Workers' Compensation Monitor of the U.S. Health Care Financing Administration and appeared in a second article in the *New York Times* (Kerr 1993b; Fig. 5). The trend toward increasing disability costs is even more evident in data from the U.S. Department of Commerce (1993) Statistical Abstracts. Temporary disability costs in the United States for 1980–90 are shown in Fig. 6, illustrating the sharply rising costs for both federal and state disability programs.

Given the obvious correlation between award of disability and costs, approximately corresponding increases in costs are expected for other industrialized countries as their numbers of patients assigned to disability status and number of medically sanctioned disability days increase. Increases in costs of health care, added to this increased utilization, can only lead to dramatic increases in overall costs of compensation programs.

The potential impact of socioeconomic factors on chronicity of low back pain, and therefore of ensuing disability awards, has been studied by Volinn, VanKoevering, and Loeser (1991). They report that in relation to short-term disability (off work 14 days or less), three types of factors double the risk of chronicity for both men and women:

Percent of 1970 Levels

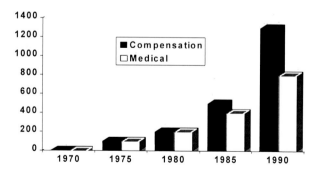

Fig. 5. Disability costs in the United States as a percentage of 1970 levels. (Kerr 1993b)

Billions of U.S. Dollars

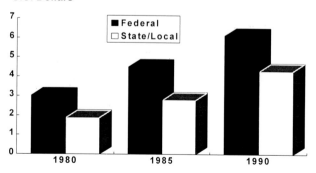

Fig. 6. U.S. federal and state temporary disability payments (in billions of dollars). (United States Department of Commerce 1993)

- *age* (claimants older than 40 years of age had twice the risk of claimants 25 years or younger)

- *monthly wage* (claimants earning $1,000 or less [in 1984] had twice the risk of claimants earning more than $2,000)

- *family status* (divorced or widowed claimants with no children had twice the risk of single claimants with no children).

Disability ascribed to low back pain has been widely perceived as a purely medical problem. Clearly, psychosocial factors loom large. The data suggest that a medical explanation is inadequate to account for the extent of the disability, and in many cases may play almost no definitive role.

THE PAIN-DISABILITY PARADOX

Melzack and Wall published the gate control theory of pain in 1965 (Melzack and Wall 1965). This seminal paper stands as a major advance in the understanding of pain and provides the underpinning to countless studies worldwide that further explicate the nature of pain. The Melzack and Wall paper presented a basis for identifying processes within the person that modulate the pain experience.

Fordyce et al. (1968a,b) reported the application of treatment methods for chronic pain based on principles and concepts derived from behavioral science. This work focused attention on the importance of interactions between the suffering person and the environment in understanding pain—a shift from attributing pain solely to pathoanatomical processes. These papers triggered numerous studies and contributed to the emergence of behaviorally based treatment programs for chronic pain.

In the ensuing decades, the profusion of research about pain has produced almost exponential growth in knowledge about the mechanisms of pain and how to measure and treat it. One might expect such decisive advances in research and knowledge to be accompanied by corresponding reductions in the magnitude of the problem of unresolved or chronic pain—including, particularly, its most expensive form: non-specific low back pain. As reported above, however, nearly the opposite is true. The incidence and prevalence of specific back pain seem to be essentially stable. And the award of disability attributed to low back pain has increased markedly and at an accelerating rate over the past several decades.

It is a paradox. Knowledge about neurophysiological, anatomical, pharmacological, and psychosocial factors implicated in back pain has advanced greatly. But the number of persons who become legally categorized as disabled from low back pain has ncreased enormously, and many remain permanently on disability rolls.

There are several reasons for the paradox. The nature of pain complaints and their relationship to suffering and mood states are not well understood by worker, employer, health care provider, and insurance and compensation agency policy maker. Methods for diagnosing and treating low back pain often are used in an ineffectual manner or are applied to problems for which they are not appropriate. Lack of technical expertise in use of diagnostic tools is not the problem; instead, it is in the conceptual basis from which pain or suffering complaints are interpreted and from which case management and treatment methods are derived. There are also defects in determination of disability, medically and legally, and in understanding complaints of back pain for which disability is being awarded. Finally, in many countries there has been a gradual shift in the concept of disability and the conditions to which it applies. The concept of disability has broadened to include matters difficult to assess and that have gone well beyond the original intent of what constitutes a compensable disability.

Back Pain in the Workplace: Management of Disability in Nonspecific Conditions, edited by W.E. Fordyce, IASP Press, Seattle, © 1995.

3

What Is Pain?

COMPLEXITY OF PAIN

Health care providers as well as persons reporting pain often do not understand the complex factors influencing complaints of pain. These misunderstandings impact diagnosis and treatment and the foundation from which insurance companies, compensation agencies, judicial systems, and employers make case decisions and set policy. To make sense of the existing chaos, it is crucial to understand pain, impairment, and disability and distinguish among them.

PAIN DEFINED

Loeser (1980) identified four dimensions to the problem of pain: nociception, pain, suffering, and pain behavior. He defines these as follows.

Nociception: potentially tissue-damaging thermal or mechanical energy impinging upon specialized nerve endings that in turn activate A-delta and C fibers.

Pain: nociceptive input to the nervous system.

Suffering: negative affective response generated in higher nervous centers by pain and other situations: loss of loved objects, stress, anxiety, etc.

Pain behavior: all forms of behavior generated by the individual commonly understood to reflect the presence of nociception, including speech, facial expression, posture, seeking health care attention, taking medications, refusing to work.

The Loeser formulation has great historical significance. As thinking has progressed, it can now be seen as perhaps too constrained in not dealing sufficiently with the social and environmental context in which pain occurs. The definitions are, however, useful in delineating critical elements in the complex phenomena of pain.

The IASP definition of pain is, "An unpleasant sensory and emotional experience associated with actual or potential tissue damage, or described in terms of such damage" (Merskey and Bogduk 1994). This definition implicates both sensory (i.e., nociception) and emotional (i.e., suffering) factors. It also draws on both "actual" and "potential" events. The definition blurs potentially observable indications of damage with unobserved descriptions when it states: "described in terms of such damage." Such a broad definition has an important role to play in providing a "flag" around which diverse approaches to the topic of pain can be rallied. As a determinative definition, it is too broad. A more detailed analysis of the concept of pain is needed.

The term *pain* is commonly used in two different and somewhat divergent ways, often without the differences being appreciated. The first refers to a signal system. Specialized nerve endings in the periphery of the body, when activated by adequate stimuli, send nerve impulses to the spinal cord or brain stem and thence onto the brain; i.e., nociception (Loeser 1980). The second use of the term lumps the signal system with cognitive, emotional, and behavioral actions occurring subsequent to nociceptive stimulation and generally conceptualized as emotions, responses, or reactions.

PAIN AS A SIGNAL

PAIN IS MORE THAN A SENSATION

The pain-as-a-signal system has elements in common with taste, smell, vision, audition, and tactile sensitivity senses; for example, specialized receptors and dedicated transmitters. However, as pointed out by Wall (1988), it does not work to categorize pain with taste, vision, smell, and tactile sensitivity as a sense. Unlike those sensory systems, pain cannot be defined independently of the response of the person experiencing it. Auditory stimulation, for example, can be identified by report or behavior of the listening person. But the stimulus and neurophysiological correlates also can be measured by analysis of an auditory signal (the sound) and by assessment of activity in the auditory nerve and brain independently of the listener's behavior in response. No such so-called objective measures currently exist for low back pain. We can know if the person is "in pain" only by his or her statements or actions. Those actions can be measured objectively, but that measurement cannot and does not assess the events that have led to their occurrence. Nociceptive impulses could theoretically be measured, but they do not define the person's responses, much less the degree of suffering. To paraphrase, in the case of most clinical pains, response measurement does not permit identification of the stimulus, and the stimulus cannot be measured.

Pain, as Wall (1988) notes, functions as a drive producing highly predictable responses comparable to hunger, thirst, and hunger for air. In the interest of preserving a stable internal environment, the person initiates complex reactions in response to such stimuli: the hungry person eats; the thirsty person drinks; the suffocating person gasps for air. Moreover, given the appropriate state of deprivation, the ameliorating response (i.e., eating, drinking, gasping) occurs in all members of the species and has a systematic relationship to the amount of deprivation (the "stimulus"). In the case of pain, however, in contrast to drive states, nociceptive stimulation may not lead to pain behaviors in different persons or at different time points or in different contextual milieus for the same person. In addition, pain carries an obligate affective component.

RELATIONSHIP OF PAIN OR SUFFERING TO NOCICEPTIVE STIMULATION

Researchers taking a neurophysiological and neuroanatomical approach have identified mechanisms that detect and transmit information about noxious stimuli to the dorsal horn of the spinal cord, and mechanisms there that receive, interpret, and transmit messages on to the brain (Bonica 1990). Others have shown, however, that no fixed relationship exists between excitation of particular afferent categories and behavioral outcomes (Wall 1988). It also has been shown that the input and output of individual

dorsal horn cells have no fixed relation. The attenuated relationship between peripheral stimulation and spinal sensory processing is, in part, a product of the plasticity of the nervous system. For example, Yaksh and Abram (1993) have stated, "Clearly, there is compelling evidence that acute afferent barrages associated with tissue trauma will generate changes in spinal sensory processing that lead to a hyperalgesic state."

The existence of hyperalgesia means that a noxious stimulus now produces an exaggerated response. Kehlet and Dahl (1993) present data indicating that "these functional changes persist for only about 80 hours." We do not know if even longer lasting changes in input-output relationships could occur. Thus, neurophysiologically and neuroanatomically based evidence indicates that pain behaviors or responses can have a variable relationship to nociceptive stimulation. Changes in the sensory processing and transmission system in response to nociceptive stimulation last but a few hours, which suggests that the effects of stimulus-driven plasticity in the nervous system are not enough in themselves to influence significantly chronic pain of many weeks' or months' duration. There is little information about plasticity engendered by environmental or affective factors influencing brain function and, thereafter, sensory processing and affective responses.

Plasticity in the central nervous system as it relates to interpretation of reports of noxious or aversive stimulation negates still further the idea that pain can be considered a simple signal system. Central nervous system responses may continue after termination of noxious stimulation, thereby compromising the inferred link between aversive stimulus and "pain" response. Moreover, pain responses may be concerned as much with impending events as with sensations, a point discussed in more detail below with regard to the role of emotions and the nature of suffering. For these reasons and others, viewing pain exclusively as a sensation or a "hard-wired" sensory system will not suffice.

PAIN AS SIGNAL PLUS ACTION

As stated above, another use of the term *pain* combines the signal system with cognitive, emotional, and behavioral actions occurring subsequent to nociceptive stimulation and generally conceptualized as emotions, responses, or reactions. These reactions, corresponding to Loeser's (1980) definitions of suffering and of pain behavior, do not occur exclusively in response to painful or nociceptive stimuli. They may occur in relation to other events unconnected with nociception, as Loeser clearly stated. They are influenced by prior experience and anticipation of consequences deriving from that experience, as well as by ambient mood state. Pain behaviors are also influenced by and may be elicited by cues indicating consequences confronting the responder.

Thus, pain behaviors are not tied exclusively to the timing of nociceptive input and, within certain variable limits, intensity of noxious stimulation.

The distinction between acute and chronic pain is also critical. Acute pain is heavily based upon the noxious stimulus, although responses are modified by age, gender, cultural, and affective factors. Chronic pain seems to have much less linkage to ongoing noxious events and much more dependence upon affective and environmental factors.

Finally, prevailing mood and "clinical" or "subclinical" nociceptive stimulation interact to influence what is perceived, how the person feels, and whether those feelings lead to the report of pain or other pain behaviors. Hearing a person complain of or describe a pain, or observing a person limping, rubbing a body part, or moving in guarded fashion, cannot be used as an absolute indicator of the presence of nociceptive stimulation. Alternative and equally viable explanations for such behaviors exist. Pain behaviors, including the verbal report of pain, should be seen as social communications and not merely as metrics of pain or nociception. Nonetheless, in the present state of affairs, disability determinations continue to be made erroneously based in substantial part, and sometimes virtually exclusively, on nothing more than observations of suffering and pain behaviors. Those are not reliable indicators of the presence of ongoing nociceptive stimuli or impairment.

THE ROLE OF EMOTIONS

The ambiguities inherent in the concept of pain relate mainly to the dynamic interplay of information reaching the central nervous system: the mixing of sensory modalities with emotional state and mood and the cognitively based anticipation of pending consequences. An aversive or nociceptive stimulus may lead to perception of pain. But active emotional states influence whether and how the aversive stimulus is perceived. Those emotional states also influence physiological processes (e.g., heart rate, blood pressure, muscle tension), which then feed back to color the perception of what is happening, the meanings assigned to it, the consequences inferred to follow, and the actions taken in response. Perception of the nature and meaning of incoming sensory information, how the body responds physiologically, and what actions are taken, as well as anticipation of what the future holds, are inextricably intertwined. We have tended to view pain as if it were a discrete element within this interactive complex of forces; it is not.

PAIN AND CARE SEEKING

Studies in industrial settings have examined factors influencing workers' rate of reporting and seeking care for symptoms. These findings, described in more detail in Chapter 6, indicate that company safety policies designed to prevent injuries from occurring have a distinct positive impact. But disability management policies conveying to workers employer concern about safety and encouraging return to work also may significantly influence symptom report and care-seeking behavior (Nachemson 1991). A worker's decision to seek care for symptoms such as pain is not automatic; it is subject to influence by a variety of factors.

Cameron et al. (1993) studied in a community-based population the decision to seek or not to seek care for a range of symptoms, including pain. They noted that "although pain may promote decisions to seek care, neither the level of pain nor perceived intensification over time seems to be a strong candidate for a determinant of care seeking." That is not to say that intensity of experienced pain cannot determine care seeking but only that other factors also influence the decision. Many hurt, but fewer perceive it as a problem for which special help is needed. A symptom may not lead to care-seeking that mandates health care.

SUFFERING

It is imperative to distinguish between pain and suffering and thus to separate pain-as-a-signal from the reactions and emotions people display when presenting to the world that they have pain. Cassell (1991) pointed out that "pain and suffering are distinct, and there can be pain (or other dire symptoms) without suffering and suffering without such symptoms." He characterizes suffering as an emotional state triggered by anticipation of threat to one's self or identity.

Budd (1992) broadened our understanding of the concept of suffering by noting that present mood state, as well as the anticipated future, influence responses to body states. He characterized suffering as occurring "when we assess ourselves in a situation and don't like where we are, where we have been, or where we are going *and* we can take no actions to close this gap." Suffering may be the ambient mood state of the person at the time the purported pain problem began or was first perceived and labeled. Alternatively, in the presence of nociceptive stimulation, mood may become suffering when anticipating what the future holds. That future may be clouded or aversive because of the anticipation of effects of perceived body damage on future functioning, whether correctly or not (Von Korff et al. 1990). However, pessimism regarding the future may occur for reasons quite unrelated to pain. Cameron et al. (1993) present further data to support this point and report that "care seekers reported more life stresses in comparison with matched controls, . . . and reported a greater number of [nonillness] life stresses in relation to the entire sample of matched controls." That implies that negatively toned mood state makes care seeking more likely. They conclude that "these findings, and the independent effect of life stressors on care seeking, are consistent with the hypothesis that care seeking will serve the critical function of reducing the load of emotional distress created both by symptoms and life stressors."

Zola (1973) studied persons seeking aid for a symptom for the first time. He concluded that "they sought help because they could not stand it any longer. But what they could not stand was more likely to be a situation or a perceived implication of a symptom rather than any worsening of the symptom *per se.*" Mood may intensify suffering to the point where the person becomes a care seeker.

JOB FACTORS

Issues within the work situation and how the worker relates to or identifies with the job are important influences on intensity of suffering and readiness to seek care for backache. Yelin and co-workers studied disabled rheumatoid arthritis patients to assess factors influencing probability that a worker will become disabled after the onset of illness (Yelin 1989). A major part of their findings is described as follows: "Control and self-employment together comprising the four best variables measuring the social characteristics of work, have an explanatory power 1.8 times as large as the four best medical, 2.2 times as large as the four best demographic, and 2.7 times as large as the four best personal resource variables." They go on to state that "workers' involvement in setting the pace of work reduces the probability that they will stop work. On the other hand, when superiors alone set the pace of work, the probability that a worker will become disabled significantly increases."

PERSONALITY AND BELIEF FACTORS

Three recently published studies lend support to this theme. Bigos et al. (1992) studied prospectively a sample from a large industrial work force, The Boeing Company, to seek predictors of back injury reports. Physical, psychosocial, and workplace factors were examined at outset of the study. Workers were followed for approximately four years, and those who reported back injury were compared on the previously accumulated assessment data with those who did not.

The study was based on data from a relatively restricted range of workers or types of jobs; namely, hourly wage workers. Moreover, depth of the ergonomic assays of jobs covered within the study was necessarily limited. These qualifications impose limits on the generalizability of study findings to different kinds of work; particularly, heavy labor and safety-sensitive jobs. Nonetheless, findings from the study raise important questions about what factors influence a worker's decision to report back pain and seek help.

Findings were as important for what they did not show as what they did. Biomechanical and ergonomic factors did not prove to be predictors of subsequent back injury report. Measures of job happiness at time of entry into the study and personality measures derived from a commonly used personality test, the

Minnesota Multiphasic Personality Inventory (MMPI; Dahlstrom et al. 1972), did. Those lower on job happiness measures were 2.5 times as likely to file back injury reports. Those with higher scores on Scale 3 of the MMPI ("Hysteria") were twice as likely to file back injury reports as those who had lower scores; however, only 14% of workers who had elevated Scale 3 scores filed back injury reports.* These findings support the concept that the existing psychological or emotional mood state exerts a significant though far from exclusive effect on care-seeking behavior and that, in the case of low back pain, ergonomic and job classification factors may be less important for many workers.

A second paper deriving from the Boeing study (Fordyce et al. 1992) analyzed in further detail data from Scale 3 of the MMPI. Scale 3 is made up of several subsets of items including descriptions of body complaints, readiness to deny social anxiety, and feelings of lassitude and malaise. The last two subsets, lassitude and malaise and denial of social anxiety, were predictive. The body complaints subset failed to differentiate those who filed back injury complaints from those who did not. Both Boeing study papers suggest that mood or psychological state may have greater predictive power, albeit modest, than do biomechanical or ergonomic measures in many work situations. At the least, these studies indicate the importance of psychosocial factors in determining who complains of pain.

Waddell and colleagues (1993) studied low back pain patients, examining relationships among measures of severity of pain, disability defined by work loss, and implications of symptoms to personal beliefs about work, activity, and cause. The best predictor of length of interval before resuming work after a reported injury was a measure of fear-avoidance beliefs about what might happen to symptoms and to underlying bodily function were work resumed. This finding further supports that the duration of disability was not uniquely linked to any of the amount of tissue damage, nociceptive activity in nerves, the conscious perception of pain, or the amount of suffering. In the

---

*Interpretation of MMPI findings in this context requires only that one recognize presence or absence of a correlation between some independent variable—in this case, filing/non-filing of a back injury claim—and an observed pattern of item responses on the test. The term *Hysteria* here connotes only the responses to a particular subset of MMPI items and has no necessary reference to the conditions sometimes called "hysteria."

Waddell study, anticipation had a greater relationship to return to work than did symptom presence or severity.

THE PHYSICIAN'S DILEMMA

An examining physician seeking to understand and treat a person presenting with the complaint of pain is faced with an ambiguous situation. The patient may not be critically or significantly different anatomically, physiologically, or psychologically from many people in the same or equivalent states who, for whatever reason, did not seek care. Diagnosis relies on information from the patient (i.e., pain behaviors), which may, unbeknownst to the patient or physician, be influenced by factors quite different from nociceptive stimulation. The process of arriving at a diagnosis is itself a complicated one. Symptoms that are not tightly linked to anatomical or physiological changes present particularly complex diagnostic problems.

DIAGNOSIS AND SPECIFICITY OR NONSPECIFICITY

Applying a diagnostic label and determining the cause of the condition are not the same. Nonspecificity of conditions, such as in nonspecific low back pain (NSLBP), means that there is not a firm and clear linkage between symptoms and diagnostic findings. Distinctions between specificity and nonspecificity of diagnosed conditions are crucial to this report. We must therefore examine the process of establishing a diagnosis. The diagnostic label provides a rationale from which treatment can be planned. It also legitimizes the relationship between an injury and the pain leading to disability. But, as has been shown in the preceding analysis of the concepts of pain and suffering, low back pain involves processes that are, by their very nature, ambiguous. This is true of both diagnosis and treatment and, therefore, also of matters of impairment and disability relating to low back pain.

The Gould Medical Dictionary defines "diagnosis" as "1. The art or the act of determining the nature of a patient's disease. 2. A conclusion reached in the identification of a patient's disease." Those definitions emphasize the judgmental nature of the diagnostic process. They also reaffirm that diagnosis and specification of causes are not the same.

Diagnosis has several functions. The obvious one

is the effort to determine the cause of symptoms to provide guidelines for treatment and management. Choice of treatment assumes there is a significant correlation between the purported causative agent and the symptoms. As a corollary, treatment plans derived from diagnosis assume that reduction or elimination of the inferred causative agent will result in reduction or elimination of symptoms. Attaching a diagnostic label subsequent to examination of a patient, however, does not establish that a substantial correlation actually exists between observed symptoms and inferred cause. Applying a diagnostic label also does not establish that ameliorating the inferred cause will lead to symptom reduction or elimination.

DIAGNOSIS AND CONCEPTUAL MODELS

The link between inferred causes and symptoms of disease is based mainly on the conceptual model from which the disease and illness are perceived. This is also true of the linkage between diagnosis and the effectiveness of treatment. Effectiveness of treatment and management can be no better than the adequacy of the conceptual model on which they are based. Low back pain should be viewed from the perspective of a biopsychosocial model of pain and illness. A biopsychosocial model is one that recognizes that symptoms—in the case of NSLBP, pain complaints—are subject to influence by factors that cannot be specified solely from anatomical or physiological parameters. The prevalent biomedical model cannot capture all of the important variables in pain behavior. The existing disability systems are all based upon a biomedical approach and must therefore be modified if we are to arrest the epidemic of disability ascribed to NSLBP.

Diagnostic labels may pinpoint causative factors; treatment of these factors can lead to reduction of symptoms. This is true of specific low back pain (which is not the subject of this report). Examples of causes of specific low back pain could be a herniated disc, metastatic cancer, or infection of the spine. When an inferred causative factor has *not* been pinpointed—as is the case with nonspecific low back pain—the diagnostic label does not reliably point to any pathophysiological change. Treatment planned from a nonspecific diagnosis often does not lead systematically to symptom reduction. In addition, of course, a diagnostic label might be accurate but the treatment prescribed may lack efficacy.

OTHER FUNCTIONS OF DIAGNOSIS

The diagnostic process may also serve other functions, some of which can distort the precision and effectiveness of treatment planning. Diagnosis may serve to rationalize to patients the treatment choices proffered by the diagnostician or therapist. Diagnosis used in that fashion is no less dependent on the adequacy of a conceptual model. The importance of an inferred substantial correlation between the alleged causative agent and symptoms, or between symptoms and the effects of planned treatment, is not diminished by applying a diagnostic label.

Diagnosis may come to serve another function in either a fee-for-service or a managed care system. Diagnosis can be manipulated by the diagnostician to ensure that proposed treatment and its charges fall within the established guidelines of the sources of authorization or reimbursement. This aspect of the diagnostic process takes on properties of legal or social engineering and has nothing to do with medical science. Diagnostic labels may become devices for sustaining professional effort or activity rather than serving as an indication for treatment. The relationship between inferred causes and symptoms and diagnosis and treatment is now burdened by selectivity of diagnostic labels in the service of reimbursement or approval actions by social or institutional mechanisms. However, the importance of the adequacy of the conceptual model remains undiminished.

Diagnostic labeling may serve yet another function. Choice of labels by the diagnostician may be tempered by judgments about what is credible or acceptable to the patient. Indeed, diagnosticians may be pressured by patients to provide diagnostic labels, however much or little confidence there may be in the labeling. This, too, can contribute to the diminished validity of a diagnosis.

Finally, attaching a diagnostic label may give the diagnostician a rationalization or greater sense of coherence for a contemplated treatment and management plan, a kind of self-reassurance, whether or not it is based on scientifically grounded findings.

These divergent functions of diagnostic labeling and treatment planning are potential forces whose importance grows when the condition being diagnosed has ambiguous properties.

NONSPECIFICITY AND THE DIAGNOSTIC PROCESS

We emphasize that low back pain is subject to influence by a variety of factors, thereby placing a particular burden on the diagnostic process. Diagnostic labels from which impairment and disability are inferred must be held accountable in terms of demonstrated specificity of alleged causes and treatment based on them. The use of specific-sounding diagnostic labels when their specificity is not demonstrated should not serve to establish presence of an impairment or a permanent disability (Hadler 1992, 1993, 1994). Impairment and permanent disability should be restricted to conditions for which causation has been demonstrated.

Failure of the health care professional or the worker complaining of pain to understand the crucial distinction between pain and suffering can be a major source of error in arriving at diagnostic labels and in disability determination proceedings. Failure of physicians to understand the distinction may lead to medically based diagnostic labels and treatment procedures having effects beyond those intended. They may solidify the worker's likely and often erroneous belief that suffering means there is something wrong for which medical intervention is needed. Failure of the worker to understand the distinction between pain and suffering leads to repeated requests or demands of the health care system to treat what is perceived as a pain problem but may be—and very often is—a problem of suffering.

BIOPSYCHOSOCIAL MODEL

Hurt and harm are not the same. To infer that suffering is to be understood, explained, and remedied by ascribing the problem exclusively to nociceptive stimulation is to start down a road that risks failure and often leads to needless persistence of suffering and disability.

For the purposes of this report we need not pursue further a more precise definition of pain. The problem addressed here is disability attributed to "pain." It is unacceptable to believe that symptoms or behaviors leading to classification as disabled by pain bear an isomorphic relationship to nociceptive stimulation or tissue damage. Disability linked to NSLBP, or to some other pain-related condition, and impairment of body function purported to relate to it, cannot be viewed solely as an expression of nociceptive stimulation.

It must be understood that the person who reports pain and is observed to be suffering, or reports suffering, is not imagining pain. Malingering (the deliberate fabrication of symptoms) is also extremely rare. The reasons for suffering, however, may not be amenable to traditional biomedically based health care. The physician and the worker reporting pain both may misconstrue suffering as indicating the need for medical intervention. Pain generally, and in NSLBP in particular, is a problem that has biological, psychological, and social aspects, all of which must be analyzed from the perspective of a biopsychosocial model (Waddell 1992).

Back Pain in the Workplace: Management of Disability in Nonspecific Conditions, edited by W.E. Fordyce, IASP Press, Seattle, © 1995.

4

Chronic Low Back Pain

AMBIGUITY IN NONSPECIFIC LOW BACK PAIN

Chronic low back pain occupies a special place in the domain of pain. One obvious reason is that people often report backache without perceiving it as a "medical" problem where the term implies that the health care system is the appropriate source for help. Conversely, the health care system frequently identifies a backache as a "medical" problem when it is not. A second reason is the ambiguity associated with back pain. A series of interlocking phenomena appear to ensure this ambiguity.

In most cases the pathoanatomical conditions underlying back symptoms remain unknown. Backache is seldom associated with clearly identifiable tissue damage or anatomical defect. That makes attributing cause a formidable task for both the professional and the suffering patient. Backache is not observable. Imaging or electrodiagnostic technology can only permit examination of structures *inferred* to contribute to or cause back pain. Lack of a systematic relationship between anatomical defects revealed on imaging and symptoms or impairment makes the task even more formidable. Finally, those who are suffering and seek help are at risk to attribute their suffering to injury. Attributing pain or suffering to injury has been a common tenet of health care systems and societies in general for many years. Backache can lead to suffering. However, suffering occurring contiguous in time to backache but minimally or not at all related to it may lead a person interpret a backache as a problem for which help is needed. As the suffering person may see it: "I am suffering and I have backache; therefore, my distress arises from back injury."

HISTORICAL PERSPECTIVE

Allan and Waddell (1989) reviewed the history of back pain, sciatica, and low back disability. They concluded (Waddell 1992):

Back pain and sciatica have affected man throughout recorded history. . . . No evidence indicates that back problems have changed. The symptom of back pain appears to be no different, no more frequent, and no more severe than it has always been.

What has changed is how back problems are understood and managed. . . . Before the nineteenth century back pain was dismissed as "fleeting pains" or rheumatics. Few became chronically disabled by simple backache. Two key ideas in the nineteenth century laid the foundations for our modern approach to back problems: (1) the pain came from the spine and (2) the pain was due to injury. . . . The physical pathology of spinal irritation was never clearly defined . . . and disappeared as a diagnosis, but the idea that the spine could be a source of pain was firmly established. The idea that a painful spine must somehow be irritable remains to this day.

The other idea was "railway spine." The building of the railways was a key part. . . . Early accidents led to a spate of serious injuries. . . . Public concern led to legislation and the start of the modern compensation system. Only then did back pain begin to be blamed on trauma. It is not easy for us to realize that, all through history, chronic back pain had never been thought to be due to injury.

TREATMENT LIMITATIONS

Several forces have contributed to the perception of backache as a medical problem for which health care system interventions have developed. Studies have not found relationships between body defect and pain, suffering, and disability; nor has the medicalization of low back pain led to solutions to the problem of incidence and prevalence of disability from backache.

Nachemson (1992) reviewed the published literature on effectiveness of prevailing treatment methods

Table 3
Proof of treatment effectiveness for NSLBP

	Duration in Days of LBP Episode			
	< 7	7–42	43–90	> 90
Bed rest < 2 days	Conclusive	Conclusive	Low	Low
Bed rest > 7 days	None	None	None	Negative
Paracetamol/NSAID	Conclusive	Conclusive	Low	Low
Manipulation	Low	High	Low	None
Back school	Low	High	Low	Negative
Heat/cold	Low	None	None	Low
Exercise (supervised)	None	Low	Conclusive	Low
Facet injection	Not applicable	Negative	Negative	Negative
Stretching	None	None	None	None
Traction	None	None	None	None
Surgery (any type)	Not applicable	None	None	None

Source: Adapted from Nachemson 1992.

for nonspecific low back pain (NSLBP). The findings reported in Table 3 indicate that the usual treatment approaches for NSLBP have failed to demonstrate significant improvement over the natural course of the condition with the few exceptions noted. Brief intervals of bed rest and selected medications are often helpful in the early days up to six weeks. Manipulation and back school may be helpful in the one- to six-week interval. Supervised exercise has demonstrated some effectiveness at six to twelve weeks. Other modalities such as facet injection, stretching, traction, and surgery have all failed to demonstrate significant benefits for NSLBP.

SUBJECTIVE INTERPRETATION OF SYMPTOMS

Examination of studies on the meaning of symptoms to the suffering person and on whether persons reporting backache seek care makes clear why there is not a systematic relationship between perceived backache and subsequent disability or functional impairment. The National Center for Health Statistics (U.S. Government, unpublished data, 1984) surveyed adult Americans regarding self-reported "major limitations" from low back pain in 1969 and again in 1981. As shown in Table 4, there was a marked increase in reported limitations in the age groups of 18–46 and older than 46 years. There is no evidence that incidence of back injury or backache had increased. These findings suggest that people, at least in the

United States, are becoming increasingly ready to describe themselves as having limitations due to low back pain.

The one-year incidence of back symptoms ranges from 27% to 60% in working adults (Frymoyer and Cats-Baril 1991; Spangfort 1988), but only 2–5% file back injury claims or seek medical care (Rousmaniere 1990; Troup et al. 1987). When is a symptom not a mandate for health care consumption? When is a "back pain problem" not a problem requiring time loss from the job?

A review of the problem of back pain in industry by Bigos and Battié (1991) makes more evident the reasons for ambiguity. They state: "Most episodes of back pain do not seem to be caused by an injury in the typical sense of the word, but rather are a normal part of life and aging. Back pain is extremely common. Up to 85% of the adult population recall having back pain by age 50, and there is some indication that the remainder have forgotten such episodes. Approximately 50% of people in the working age group admit to significant symptoms but only a small percentage (2–5%) subsequently make the decision to file a back

Table 4
Major limitations from self-report of low back pain

	Rate per 100,000 by Age Group		
Year	18–46	46+	All
1969	98	365	192
1981	210	750	394

Source: National Center for Health Statistics, unpublished data, 1984.

injury claim. Furthermore, only about one-fifth of patients with back problems can loosely associate the onset of their symptoms with an accident, injury or unusual activity."

The observations of Bigos and Battié, and the supporting studies they cite, show the ambiguities inherent in the complaint of low back pain, and reaffirm that something more is involved in the problem than nociceptive stimulation. A small percentage of those who report onset of back pain in work settings and perceive the problem as warranting medical care, can identify some event as a cause of onset.

Clearly, in work-related back pain reports selective factors exert influence from the outset to determine whether a person decides perceived backache warrants seeking care. Battié (1992) reviewed the professional literature on worksite interventions to reduce disability from back pain, including but not restricted to NSLBP, a subject discussed in Chapter 6. She states: "The investigator is aware of no studies demonstrating that strength, flexibility, or aerobic capacity play a significant role in back pain reporting in occupations of light or moderate physical demands."

Another cost-related effect of disability for NSLBP concerns the probability of return to work once work has ceased and medical help has been sought. Waddell (1992) has calculated the probability of return to work based on data from several studies. The findings reported in Fig. 7 suggest that the probabilities of ever returning to work diminish sharply if an early return to work does not occur, falling below 50% in six months.

Review of studies of the effects of worksite-based prevention programs on care-seeking for back pain and on subsequent disability rates lends more support for questioning the state of the back as the defining factor in back pain (Hunt and Habeck 1993). These studies suggest a greater impact on reduction of back pain–related disability rates from policies and programs not involving medical interventions designed to modify the state of the spine or back musculature. Changes in disability rates are not the same as changes in intensity of back pain; the report of back pain is not an index of ability to work.

AGE AND GENDER

This section examines age and gender in relation to occurrence and persistence of NSLBP, primarily in

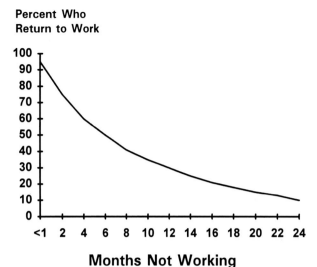

Percent Who Return to Work

Months Not Working

Fig. 7. Probability of return to work in relation to months off work. (Adapted from Waddell 1992)

persons of working age. The data reported do not permit differentiating specific from nonspecific low back pain.

Raspe (1993) in his review of the international professional literature, cited in Chapter 2, concluded that there is no unequivocal influence of age on incidence of back pain. The survey of compensated back injury in Quebec, Canada (Spitzer et al. 1987), describes age and gender incidence patterns for low back pain as measured by workers who filed compensation claims for temporary disability. Those data focus on a working population and show higher rates of incidence in younger age groups. Higher rates for men occur in the 15–19 and 20–24 age brackets. Rates for women are low in the 15–19 age group, peak in the 20–24 group and then, as with men, decrease in succeeding age groups (Fig. 8).

Mayer et al. (1991) report prevalence of low back pain complaints in a geographical area sampling from Vermont in the United States. A sample of the general population showed a slight tendency for men to have greater prevalence beyond age 65 than in earlier years, followed by men aged 25–35 years, and a slight reduction through the middle years. In moderate contrast, women showed a slightly greater prevalence from 35–45 with a tendency for the rate to diminish in subsequent years. Incidence rates are clearly higher in men over women in the younger (15–19, 20–24) age groups. Thereafter, gender differences diminish with age. The prevalence rates shown in Fig. 9 indicate few gender differences, and those occur mainly in older, non-working-age persons.

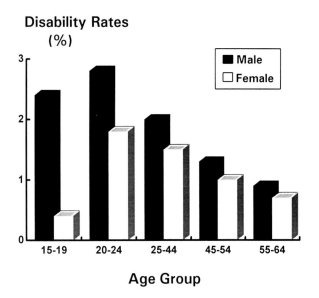

Fig. 8. Disability rates (%) for NSLBP by age and gender among Canadian workers who filed compensation claims for temporary disability. (Spitzer et al. 1987)

The Nuprin Pain Report, a survey of adult Americans (Taylor and Curran 1985), indicates that the percentage who report backache in the past year drops with age: 63% of those 18–24 report one or more backaches compared with 49% of those over age 65. However, backache is clearly more of a chronic problem in the older age group: 16% reporting backaches for more than 101 days, compared with 6% of those aged 18–24 years.

The Nuprin report (Taylor and Curran 1985) also states that women are only slightly more likely to report having had backache in the past year than are men: 57% vs. 53%, a negligible difference. In addition, the report suggests that working mothers are no more likely than homemakers (58% vs. 56%) to have experienced backaches in the past year.

Walsh et al. (1992) studied prevalence of back pain and associated time off work in eight areas of Britain. Their findings, reported in Table 5, indicate no appreciable differences in prevalence between males and females. The findings also indicate a tendency for males to be off work longer than females in younger (20–39) years but this difference disappears in the 40–49 age group, only to reappear in the 50–59 age bracket.

The study by Walsh and co-workers dealt only with age ranges from 20–59. Their findings roughly approximate those found in the United States by Mayer et al. (1991; Fig. 8) in that among men prevalence tends to increase with age. In contrast, women showed a one-year prevalence peaking between ages 40–49 (43.7%) and then diminishing in the 50–59 age bracket (35.7%).

The Mayer et al. (1991) and Nuprin (Taylor and Curran 1985) studies reported data from the United States, Spitzer et al. (1987) studied a Canadian population, and Walsh et al. (1992) investigated workers in Great Britain. Their findings are similar with regard to both age and gender factors. Raspe's (1993) review of the international professional literature yielded comparable findings.

Overall, the findings reported here indicate that incidence of back pain reports is greater in the

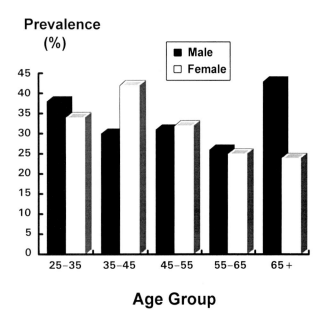

Fig. 9. Prevalence (%) of low back pain by age and gender in a sample of Vermont residents. (Mayer et al. 1991)

Table 5
Prevalence of back pain and time off work
in workers in eight areas of Britain

| | Prevalence of Back Pain (%) by Age Group | | | |
	20–29	30–39	40–49	50–59
Men				
Back pain	35.4	37.1	38.2	40.5
Off work	9.5	13.5	9.4	9.5
Women				
Back pain	27.0	33.6	43.7	35.7
Off work	6.1	5.1	9.8	6.5

Source: Data from Walsh et al. 1992.

younger men but not women. Younger men tend to be involved in more physically demanding activities, whether at work or play. However, studies of progressively older men show no systematic increase in incidence or in persistence of back pain and associated disability until 50 years and older. Lower rates among men in the middle years could indicate that severe back injuries in earlier years led more back-vulnerable workers to withdraw from vigorous work.

The probable history of having engaged in more vigorous activities at work and play in the earlier years may contribute to cumulative effects and more back pain in later years, whether a person is still in the labor force or retired. Higher rates in older men may be related to increased rate of suffering for whatever reason, pain or otherwise.

Incidence and prevalence among women is different, as are their probable histories for the extent of involvement in physically vigorous activities. Women have not shown an increase in back pain with increasing age beyond the middle years.

Several conclusions can be drawn from these data that are of particular importance to laws and policies bearing on long-term disability from NSLBP. First, prevalence of persisting NSLBP appears to have at most a slight relationship to age during the working years. Incidence of NSLBP-related events may be higher in younger men, but without greater persistence into chronicity. Therefore, the age factor may be of little consequence among men until after retirement. Second, in women, incidence and prevalence have a complex relation to age: less in younger and older samples, more in middle-age.

Third, differences in age patterns of incidence between men and women and the lack of differences among women who are working vs. homemakers suggests that persisting dysfunction from low back pain is not tied closely to age until the near-retirement years and then, if at all, in men only. Does this mean that greater prevalence of back pain among men reflects a cumulative effect of participation in more physically vigorous work-related activity? If that were true, we would expect a trend toward increasing amounts of time off work from back pain events in later working years. The Walsh et al. (1992) data, as reported in Table 5, indicate otherwise; i.e., there was no reported increase in amount of time off work from back pain as a function of age. If the increased prevalence of back pain in retirement-aged men is to be ascribed to cumulative effects of employment, these data should be different.

MEDICALIZATION OF SUFFERING

The absence of clear age or gender incidence and prevalence patterns suggests that back pain-related disability relates more to other factors than to age or gender. The data do not permit separation of specific from nonspecific causes of low back pain, but the preponderance of the latter suggests that NSLBP has the same age and gender-related characteristics.

For both logical and empirical reasons we may question whether back pain complaints in industrial settings are automatically a problem requiring or relevant to medical care. The analysis and discussion of pain and suffering in Chapter 3 pointed out how easily the two are confounded by both patients and medical professionals. Suffering, when misattributed to nociception and pain, usually leads to efforts to remediate the problem by medical means; the major problem in NSLBP disability appears to be the medicalization of suffering.

Back Pain in the Workplace: Management of Disability in Nonspecific Conditions, edited by W.E. Fordyce, IASP Press, Seattle, © 1995.

5

Impairment and Disability

The concepts of impairment and disability require close examination to understand the conceptual bases of existing approaches to disability management.

DISABILITY PROGRAM INTENT

The concept of disability can be traced back to medieval times (Mendelson 1988; Spangfort 1988). The "whole person" concept was the guiding principle. Historically, "whole person" referred to intactness of the body. Injury resulting in loss of some body part or function led to efforts to restore that person as closely as possible to the "whole person" inferred to have existed prior to injury. Disability benefit and workmen's compensation programs were first established by Bismarck in Germany more than a century ago (Mendelson 1988; Spangfort 1988) to provide assistance in restoring an injured worker to competitive opportunity. As noted by Berkowitz and Berkowitz (1991), "the worker was not supposed to benefit from the accident, but was entitled to a cash amount designed to preserve living standards." Workmen's compensation and other disability benefit programs continue within that frame of reference.

What is intended in providing support for disabled persons and their families? Disability benefit programs provide the person with resources that can help regain access to competitive opportunity in the working world, a concept of temporary assistance. In the event of an irremediable condition, a partial economic haven may be provided for the employee and family in lieu of work; a status implying permanent disability or partial disability with or without potential for work. The commitment of part of finite social resources for managing the problem of disability must inevitably have limitations.

THE BROADENING OF THE DISABILITY CONCEPT

Based on the "whole person" concept, loss of listed body parts, or their becoming irremediably nonfunctional for competitive employment, could lead to assessment of impairment and, subsequently, the award of disability. In the past century the concept of disability gradually broadened (Mendelson 1988; Spangfort 1988) to incorporate physiological and psychological processes as potential factors for evaluation and, where indicated, remediation. This broadening reflects the effects of several evolving factors. One is improvement in societal resources for providing discretionary support for those unable to assume fully productive roles. A second is the decreasing role of the family as an agency of social welfare. A third is the expansion of knowledge leading to a greater awareness of the inseparability of mind and body and, correspondingly, of the concept of what constitutes "the whole person." There is, as well, a generally greater capability for the remediation of dysfunction of whatever type.

The impetus for broadening the definitions of work-related conditions to be considered as disabling also comes in part from the health care system proffering remedies even when they have questionable links to the conditions they are purported to treat. Health care professionals lay claim to diagnostic and restorative capability for an ever-widening array of conditions. Demonstrated correlations between pathoanatomical findings and functional performance and the probability that interventions will restore normal function may be marginal or lacking. Even so, that often does not diminish the enthusiasm with which health care is recommended.

On the other side is the suffering worker. Whatever the cause of suffering, medically based diagnostic categories and treatment programs are there to be called upon. Worker demand for remedies for suffering provides further reinforcement to professionals seeking to help. The result is a broadening of expectations by both health care purveyors and workers.

An axiom from behavioral science applies here: if a behavior persists it *is* being reinforced. If assignment to or receipt of persisting disability status is increasing in the absence of evidence of corresponding increases in injury rates, we must ask why? Whose interests are being served? To what extent do professionals, stimulated in part by consumer demand, resort to diagnoses and treatment methods derived from dubiously valid disease-model-based ideas? To what extent is growing consumer demand a product of increasing reliance on medically based solutions to life problems fueled in part by health care system "promises" of remedy? To what extent does increasing demand result from increasing acceptance of medically sanctioned disability status as an alternative to extant suffering, however much or little that suffering is related to work injury?

A broadened view of what constitutes a disability places a new burden on disability management. Impairment-rating-based disability programs assume and require a measurable performance deficit linked to pathoanatomy. This proposition is subject to challenge (e.g., Hadler 1992, 1993). The scope and persistence of symptoms, perhaps only loosely related to pathoanatomy, often may be changed by interventions that do not alter pathoanatomy. Broadening the base of compensable deficit to include performance deficits not attributable to pathoanatomical impairment changes the basis for the determination of disability. The "whole person" concept in its historical meaning can no longer serve as the defining base if non-anatomical and nonphysiological functions subject to influence or control by factors outside the person are included in disability determination. Insofar as they have been, the result is the disability epidemic that this report addresses.

The precise scope of conditions to which disability benefits may apply varies from society to society and among programs within each society. The general principle, however, based on the "whole person" concept, has been to use a disease model to define conditions and their management. It is an impairment-rating paradigm. A better balance between disability-related desires of the individual and the needs of society must be found.

BENEFITS AS OPPORTUNITY, NOT GUARANTEE

Embedded in the concept of disability are two implicit principles that are not always recognized and understood. One is that disability benefits are intended to provide opportunity to compete; not to provide guarantees that competitive effort will always succeed. The contract between a society and an individual for disability benefits presumably intends to optimize opportunity for success when disability has resulted in a performance or competitive disadvantage. To guarantee success to its individual members, a society would have to commit resources in an open-ended manner. The history of soaring disability costs relating to nonspecific low back pain (NSLBP) illustrates the adverse effects of such a course.

To imply guaranteed restoration of function or, in the presence of dysfunction, a near-as-possible equivalency of the economic fruits of function, has effects on the individual as well as on society. In a capitalistic society, economic and social competitiveness gain special emphasis that influences motivation toward the economic and social rewards of employment. Work often becomes the major focus of a person's efforts to achieve material rewards and life's pleasures. For some it becomes a raison d'être. Disability policy which, however inadvertently, serves to diminish that raison d'être can have detrimental effects on health and well-being that are beyond any intended effects.

When workers perceive that a claim for work-related injury can result in equivalent social and economic reward, their motivation to return to work can be compromised. When a worker submits a claim for disability, there is often an expectation of a guarantee that either the health care system will restore the individual to normal function or there will be compensation that provides approximately equal income in the face of a permanent disability. The worker often does not perceive that the guarantee is for, as much as possible, a "level playing field" for access to personal and family health.

Success, given a level playing field of opportunity, will depend upon individual performance. As in all of life, performance will be exposed to the exigencies of mischance that may result in failure; e.g., failures of the economy, failures of the employing company, failures of the worker's family to permit or adequately support sustained effort during or subsequent to rehabilitative efforts. Those exigencies arise from events in the environment that are external to the concept of the "whole person."

THE IMPORTANCE OF WORKER EFFORT

Failure at work may arise from insufficient worker effort or from inadequate coping with work demands or the social milieu of the worksite. Those are reasons not attributable to loss or impairment of body parts. "Effort-related" matters have special importance to the social contract between an individual and society. They provide, or intend to provide, certain opportunities and benefits. But those opportunities and benefits cannot exist on a noncontingent basis. The person has obligations, as does society. Society's opportunities and benefits cannot exist without individual contribution or effort. Societies may provide specific exclusion from this part of the social contract, but the extent to which they can do so must have limits.

The capacity of disability programs to remediate matters not firmly rooted in pathoanatomical factors is central to the problem now being addressed. The "exigencies of mischance," as they were paraphrased above, are matters of interest and importance to society and should also be addressed, though not in the context of this report. Important factual and conceptual issues provide a basis for challenging the adequacy and the practicality of the broadened "whole person" perspective as a method of dealing with disability as pertains to pain, particularly NSLBP.

THE LOGIC OF IMPAIRMENT
AND DISABILITY

A second implicit principle in the concept of disability is that the disability determination process makes judgments. Impairment is judged to be potentially remediable or not. In the former case, remediation programs make up part of the process of rehabilitation of the disabled. Disability benefits are intended to assist the person and the family unit on a temporary basis while remediation is under way; societies provide resources to assist. If remediation is not an option, permanent disability benefits may be available. The extent to which each society provides such benefits of course varies.

Disability programs have generally been applied based on a logic that holds that body processes, including symptoms, can ultimately be explained by understanding underlying anatomical or physiological mechanisms. It is a biological reductionistic model and a "top-down" logic in which phenomena such as symptoms are seen as causally related to body processes. It is also a mind-body dualism model implying that mind and body are separable entities, each exerting influence on the other. However, it has long been recognized that mind and body processes inseparably influence function. One does not "cause" the other or direct it. Instead, they interact in a dynamic and often proactive way. Body defects or aberrations influence the mind and the person's interpretation of and anticipations about the environment in which he or she is functioning. Conversely, personal attitudes and expectations as well as environmental influences help to shape and modulate the impact of body processes on functioning. This interaction is more than the simple sum of its parts. Concepts of impairment and disability must consider this dynamic interaction and not underestimate the extent to which cognitive and mental processes influence body processes, and vice versa.

Response to an impairment and the extent to which alternative activities are pursued are shaped by individual effort as well as by opportunity. That effort draws not only on anatomical and physiological mechanisms, but also on cognitive or mental processes. The meanings or expectations generated in the person by the situation, and the environmentally rooted consequences of effort, are critical.

SIDE-EFFECTS OF A DISEASE
MODEL PERSPECTIVE

Mind-body dualism as applied to the determination of impairment and disability can lead to another pitfall. The perception of anatomical or physiological defects isolated from environmental factors risks casting the person into a role as passive recipient of a performance disadvantage both in the eyes of the health care professional and the injured worker. The body (and the mind) tend to be perceived as fixed entities which, when damaged, require repair. Viewing the body as an "inert recipient" of injury has similarities to viewing a macadam road that accumulates pits and chuckholes with use. Remediation awaits road repair crews just as the person injured may await restoration from the health care system. That view is to be contrasted with, for example, an athlete who, on sustaining an injury, may respond by increased effort so as better to stimulate healing processes and to maintain or regain function in the face of impairment and distress. The increased effort may be self-initiated or as a result of prompting and encouragement from others, including health care professionals. The success of such efforts is dependent, of course, on type and severity of the injury. The point is that people are not inert or in a fixed state of being. They are dynamic organisms having the potential for contributing to self-restoration of structure and function by the actions they take.

There is a further risk when the health care system is perceived as the responsible agent for fixing matters. Anything increasing the injured worker's self-perception as a passive recipient of health care can have a stifling effect on patient effort. This factor is perhaps the major hidden cost of the broadened concept of disability.

Processes by which disability is defined and diagnosed create expectations in health care professionals and injured workers alike. Insofar as those expectations assign principal responsibility for remediation to the professional, a double loss may follow. The professional may continue to emphasize ineffectual remediation efforts, thereby needlessly exposing the worker to the adverse effects of protracted disability. In doing so there may also be a failure to encourage patient effort. The worker, in turn, may look to the professional for remediation rather than to his/her own efforts as a major factor determining outcome.

This passive "role casting" tends to absolve the disability determination process from considering the full range of alternative ways to influence the ability to perform. It overlooks the importance of individual effort in determining whether and to what extent disability is present. This analysis of the logic underlying impairment and disability highlights the influence of environmental and cognitive/mental processes on human performance and on healing and the restoration of function.

CONCEPT OF IMPAIRMENT

The World Health Organization (WHO) has defined impairment as "any loss or abnormality of psy-

chological, physiological, or anatomical structure or function" (1980). Body injury may result in an impairment. Subsequent performance of the person determined disabled is, however, subject to influence by factors beyond those defined by the impairment.

Generally, impairment refers to loss of body function, as when a limb is amputated, a stroke results in hemiparesis, or spinal cord injury leads to paraplegia. If the condition is remediable, impairment may be temporary. Amputation of an upper extremity influences the ability to screw on a jar lid or to play a clarinet. However, the amputee may acquire adaptive equipment to assist in opening jars and exert the necessary effort to master and use them. The person may have an impairment but is he or she disabled with respect to jar opening? The answer is, of course, "no," but not only because there are multiple ways to screw on jar lids but also because performance ultimately is influenced by personal effort and determination. The clarinetist may no longer be able to play the clarinet, or virtually any other musical instrument, but is precluded from engaging only in productive activities requiring bimanual function.

Disability, considered in more detail below, is defined as "any restriction or lack of the ability to perform an activity in the manner or within the range considered normal for a human being" (World Health Organization 1980; Snook and Webster 1987). In an impairment-rating paradigm, assignment of permanent disability is contingent upon presence of an associated impairment.

Performance of a person to whom an impairment is ascribed does not have an isomorphic relationship to a body defect, anatomical or physiological (e.g., Hadler 1992, 1993). Not all potential impairments can be confirmed by verifiable measures of their presence independent of performance by the person purported to be impaired. Because performance is also "effort-related" as well as related to anatomical or physiological capabilities, it is inevitably linked to and influenced by such factors as attitudes, motivation and personality. They in turn are inextricably linked to consequences in the perceived immediate or the anticipated environment. Those factors are the person/environment interactions and not simply characteristics of the person.

Perception and interpretation of environmental cues and environmental feedback regarding performance generate expectancies that in turn influence attitudes, motivation, and personality, and the behaviors which ensue. These factors play critical roles in pain behaviors. The relationship of pain behaviors, a central part of NSLBP, to environmental influences is particularly great. For example, Romano et al. (1991) documented that spouse response to patient pain behavior may influence the subsequent frequency of expressions of those behaviors. Performance relating to anatomical or physiological defects does not have a "stand-alone" character capable of being singled out as an impairment and from that a disability. Performance also is wedded to the environment. It should be obvious that sufficient "effort" can not always overcome every impairment.

ANATOMICAL DEFECTS

Defining impairment from the presence of anatomical defects requires certain assumptions. Human anatomy is not static; it is ever changing, though often slowly. In the case of NSLBP and its related anatomical structures, bony changes in the spine are associated with aging. These progressive spinal changes illustrate the necessity of recognizing that such concepts as "normal" and "abnormal" can be defined with respect to anatomical structures only in relative terms. Moreover, there is a variable correlation and not a 1:1 relationship between anatomical structure and behavioral function. Anatomical structures may or may not be influenced by immediate or short-term environmental influences; similarly, effects of performance or behavior relating to them may be variable. Long-term participation in physically vigorous activities may produce measurable change in, for example, spinal anatomical structures. Those changes can be verified by imaging techniques rather than effort-related performance by the patient. However, the extent of their influence on performance is variable.

The changing character of anatomical structures complicates the definition of impairment based on anatomical features. A beginning is to limit definition of permanent impairment based on anatomical defects to states definable independently of behavior, as being irremediable, and as having objectively verifiable interference in function. Presence of an anatomical defect by so-called "objective" measures (i.e., measures not based on effort-related patient behavior) should be seen as necessary but not sufficient to define impairment. Definition of impairment should require a clearly established link between the particular structural defect or degenerative condition and symptoms or performance.

Definition of impairment based on anatomical factors should also require consideration of appropriate age and history issues. Finally, its definition should occur with the full recognition that patient performance may be little correlated with anatomical structure. Qualified health care professionals, assuming they consider the dynamic character of anatomical structures and use appropriate evaluative procedures, should be capable of determining an anatomical basis for impairment. However, having done so does not establish disability.

PHYSIOLOGICAL STATES

The definition of impairment may also be based on presence of purportedly abnormal physiological states inferred to influence performance. Physiological states have an even more complex relationship to environmental events than do anatomical factors. Some physiological states are reflexive in nature. Physiological reflexes may be cued by the environment; e.g., increased heart rate when threat is perceived. When they persist at abnormal levels, if not remediable by medically based interventions (e.g., pharmacological or surgical), they can meet the standard of permanent impairment. Moreover, extended exposure to environmental forces can result in lasting changes in physiological functions even after those adverse environmental forces are no longer present. That point is particularly pertinent to pain (Price 1986; Wall 1988). Wall (1988) hypothesizes: "The classical assumption has been that pain would only continue so long as there was a continuous source of nociceptive impulses in the periphery. With the discovery of at least three different types of central control system, it is necessary to consider the possibility that peripheral pathology could trigger an abnormal resetting of the central controls so that pain persists after the original peripheral signal has ceased."

Physiological states caused by persisting but now absent environmental effects and judged by competent evaluation to be abnormal can be considered as potential impairments if remediation to normal ranges is not possible. How much those states result in inability to perform is a separate matter to be determined.

Physiological states can have strong links to continuing environmental effects. Of many possible examples, a few will illustrate a spectrum of physiological processes that are sensitive to environmental effects and have enduring consequences. Redd (1980) demonstrated environmental stimulus control in the form of selective nurse responses to nausea and retching in acute leukemia patients. As long ago as 1955, Jarvinen (1955) reported that patients hospitalized with myocardial infarction were five times as likely to experience sudden death when unfamiliar staff were making ward rounds. Engel et al. (1974) demonstrated that conditioning paradigms could enhance discrimination of rectal pressure, leading to an often successful method of treating rectal incontinence. Kaplan and Hartwell (1987) showed a significant effect on physiological parameters of patients with type II diabetes mellitus from differential social support and social networks.

These examples imply that physiological processes ought not to be seen automatically as "stand-alone" states. They have, or potentially have, significant links to the person's environment. Physiological states implicating the environment differ in their relationship to definitions of impairment. Lasting changes in physiological processes resulting from prolonged exposure to adverse environmental influences, if identifiable by competent medical evaluation independent of effort-related patient behavior, meet the criteria for impairment. However, these aberrant physiological processes do not necessarily result in disability; nor are they pain. Persisting physiological states based on remediable environmental influences should be seen as remediable temporary disability states and not as permanent impairments.

PSYCHOLOGICAL FACTORS

A key element in understanding the role of psychological factors in impairment and disability is to recognize that human behavior has an often underappreciated link to the environment. Humans demonstrate lasting and pervasive ways of behaving that appear to have virtual independence from immediate environmental influence. Compulsive persons may behave in compulsive ways across time and a spectrum of situations. Highly anxious or depressed persons may display persisting signs of anxiety or depression in many situations or environments. Those are extreme examples and even they do not show total independence from the environment.

The influence on behavior of expectancies from environmental feedback has major implications for definitions of impairment and disability. This is particularly true where anatomical or physiological impairment has not been demonstrated independently of the effort-related activity of the person.

Lee (1992) stated, "The traditional distinction between behavior (or organism) and environment obscures the transdermal nature of acts. This formulation conceptualizes acts as units that have organismic and environmental constituents and not as units located exclusively in the organism." Powers (1973) notes, "All behavior involves strong feedback (environmental interaction) effects, whether . . . spinal reflexes or self-actualization. It is (so) all pervasive and fundamental . . . it is as invisible as the air we breathe." These comments highlight the relational basis of behavior to environment. They interact, each influencing the other. Behavior should not be viewed independently of its interactions with the environment.

Psychological aspects of impairment involve personality and behavior. Inferences about "personality" are derived largely from a person's behavior. This approach does not imply that psychological aspects of impairment and of disability involve only behavior, simply that we cannot safely ignore the behavioral components. A person may show significant psychological dysfunction persisting in many environments or social contexts and across time.

Psychological functions pertinent to disability determination should not be assessed independently of the associated environmental factors. We lack "objective" evaluation tools or procedures that are effective irrespective of the environmental context of behavior and that are independent of a person's effort. Moreover, impact of psychological impairments on behavior varies with the particular set of tasks. The effect of an upper extremity amputation is likely to be felt in all activities involving bimanual function. Extreme hypertension or persisting cardiac irregularities may influence virtually all of the person's performance repertoire. Psychological impairment resulting from, for example, a childhood of severe parental physical abuse and leading to pervasive anxiety, may be followed in subsequent years by performance difficulties, but which ones and in what ways is likely to be influenced greatly by the immediate context.

Psychological impairments have virtually an inevitable environmental link. The "effort-related" dimension to human performance can never be addressed independently of environmental factors. Incentives and consequences anticipated by the person may have major influence on performance pertaining to psychological impairments. Central to the point of this report, abnormal psychological functions are not "pain."

THE SOCIAL CONTRACT AND PSYCHOLOGICAL IMPAIRMENT

Consideration of psychological impairments involves the social contract between the individual and society. As noted previously, societies may provide benefit programs designed to enhance a person's opportunity to compete, though they cannot guarantee success. Such programs are likely to draw in part on two assumptions that need to be examined and understood: namely, that people are somewhat equal with respect to their potential for "success," and that sufficient effort by social programs that can remedy inequalities. Both assumptions are untenable.

Earlier, in introducing this issue, the term "exigencies of mischance" was used to point out that success cannot be guaranteed. Failure to succeed (at, for example, a job or a rehabilitation program) does not occur randomly owing to the whims of a capricious world. People enter the world of work with varying repertoires and potentials. Some are strong, some weak. Some are bright, others not so bright. Some have backgrounds equipping them with self-confidence and effective problem-solving and social-coping skills. Others, products of a less favorable childhood environment, may be less well prepared for the world of work and for dealing with the "exigencies of mischance." Failure is more likely to occur in those with less effective repertoires. Disability management policy should take that into account. Societies vary in their ability to provide remediation, particularly in regard to psychological problems. Societies also vary in how much they can or will commit in resources to minimize the impact of these inequities of ability to participate in work and other activities.

A given society may decide to exempt persons with one or more forms of impairment from the obligation of participating in work and productive effort. Examples might be persons with profound mental retardation, congenital defects such as blindness or spina bifida, or congenitally malfunctioning cardiovascular systems and other physiological defects. To what extent would exemptions be given for those with severe psychological problems deriving from, for example, childhood abuse where effects on function will vary from person to person and work situation to work situation? It is a choice each society must make. The choice should be tempered by capabilities for remediation and by the extent to which changes in the environment or milieu can lead to significant amelioration. It should also be tempered by the extent to which individual effort irrespective of or in conjunction with a remediation program can influence the outcome. Those are social and political or public policy choices.

In granting an exception to the obligation to engage in productive activity society is saying, in effect, that "If you have (whatever dysfunction) and our capabilities for overcoming that dysfunction are insufficient to permit you to participate in gainful employment, you are absolved from the responsibility of seeking and holding a job." But this stance raises another issue. Is being "absolved" from work to be dealt with by classification as impaired, with whatever social and monetary benefits may accrue to that, including, in some societies, access to health care pertinent to the impairment? That is one logical choice. However, that choice carries with it special burdens for society and the taxpayer. It exposes the person to health care treatments and costs specific to the impairment. In addition, the health care system tends to convey to the person that the dysfunction is subject to remediation by that system whether true or not, and that "effort-related" contributions to restoration of function may not be crucial, or even helpful. That choice also provides a potent environmental reinforcer to remain on disability status: the fear of the loss of health care funding.

Another social/political option is assignment as unemployed (presumably, unemployable). The social and political or public policy issue in this case concerns the extent to which society provides support for maintenance of the person and his/her family unit by unemployment benefits. Assignment as unemployed should occur when it is not possible to restore or create "equality" sufficient to permit engaging in gainful employment. Psychological problems, for example, should not be seen as pain problems. If impairment or disability status is to be awarded, it should be for the psychological problems. Decisions as to the range and type of psychological problems for which impairment and subsequent disability benefits might be provided are important matters but beyond the scope of this report. We have chosen to focus on NSLBP, for there is clear evidence that present policies are failing to come to grips with core issues, leading to increasing costs, both social and financial.

JOB STRESS

Psychological problems enter into disability management considerations in another way. Worksite difficulties can lead to suffering. Performance demands of the job may be stressful or beyond the capabilities of the worker. Interpersonal difficulties within the social milieu of the worksite may be stressful and lead to emotional disturbance. There are many other possible examples. Extent and duration of suffering will be influenced by intensity of the sources of stress at the worksite. They will also be influenced by the coping skills of the worker and by the extent to which, as with "physical injury," the worker takes positive action to maintain or restore function. An even more basic point is that there are better alternatives during remediation of job dysfunction than defining the problem as impairment and, from that, disability. Social programs to provide assistance in searching for employment better fitted to the person's stress/coping resources offer one such alternative.

TEMPORARY AND PERMANENT DISABILITY

Permanent disability status should require that the condition exists independently of the environment in which the person functions. A person may have an impairment, but unless there are anatomical, physiological, or psychological defects measurable independently of effort-related job performance and the environmental influences on that performance, the conclusion should not be a permanent disability. Abnormality of anatomical structure that in turn significantly influences performance and that is deemed irremediable may qualify as an impairment. Simple fracture of an arm bone impairs function during healing time and a brief period of rehabilitation, but barring complications of the healing, not thereafter.

Abnormality from a physiological function with a limited relation to the environment may qualify as an impairment. Disease processes with known links to neurophysiological defects such as multiple sclerosis or muscular dystrophy also can qualify as impair-

ments. Physiological abnormalities linked to long-term exposure to environmental influences and judged to be irremediable can be measured independently of patient behavior, and are potentially determinable as impairments. Abnormality from physiological function linked to potentially remediable environmental factors is not an impairment, though it may lead to temporary disability status.

Psychological dysfunction, psychotic or otherwise, is not a measure of pain and should not be attributed to nociceptive stimulation. Appropriately qualified psychiatric or psychological assessment should suffice to determine presence of psychological dysfunction. However, the complaint of pain should not be the basis for such determination, even though psychological dysfunction may have been initiated by a pain problem or by job-related stress. Permanent pain-related disability status derived from psychological dysfunction should not be assigned as a part of a disability program. Each society must decide whether such psychological distress related to the job should be considered a compensable work-related injury. Determination of that issue should consider whether the condition is remediable, whether changes in the work environment to ameliorate the problem are reasonably attainable (see Chapter 6 for further consideration of these issues), and responsibilities of the worker to influence restoration of function.

To summarize, anatomical, physiological, or psychological abnormalities sufficient to limit performance may qualify as impairments, though not necessarily as pain-related, if they are measurable independent of effort-related performance and if they are not readily modifiable by direct treatment interventions or by addressing the interaction between performance and environment. "Specific" back pain is potentially an impairment only to the extent that it adversely affects (impairs) function; that is, the pain-related impairment is the restriction or limitation of movement (as per the WHO definition) and not pain per se.

We present this rather detailed consideration of the concept of impairment because of its deep roots in our ways of thinking about disability. However, recognition of the potential impact of remediation and environmental modifications on performance makes clear that the concept of impairment is not a reasonable basis for determining disability due to NSLBP. Impairment-rating based disability programs does not meet the needs of society and is leading to an under-mining of benefit programs.

DISABILITY

The WHO definition of disability is: "any restriction or lack (resulting from an impairment) of the ability to perform an activity in the manner or within the range considered normal" (1980).

If the concept of impairment—and its definition—cannot be applied to chronic NSLBP without considering the environmental context of the person, then disability, too, cannot be applied without implicating the environment. Thus, there are problems with the WHO definition of disability.

A person reporting persisting pain can be presumed to be suffering. That suffering may involve nociceptive stimulation. But it may also involve other unpleasant mood states or emotional distress. Failure to recognize the potential divergence of nociceptive stimulation and reported pain or suffering leads to unwarranted assignment of disability status.

Yelin (1989) addressed the concept of disability. He said:

> The word disability is used to connote the presence of illness, reduced capacity to function, an actual reduction in functioning, and handicap. Largely due to the failure to distinguish among these concepts, researchers have developed discrete terms for each step in a process which begins with the onset of injury or disease and proceeds to an actual change in function. Thus, pathophysiological changes may occur in the body, even prior to being noticed by the individual as a symptom; when such changes occur a disease is onset. The autoimmune changes which much later result in rheumatoid arthritis are an example. After onset, the disease may affect the body's physical processes. Rheumatoid arthritis limits the range of motion of joints, Alzheimer's disease affects cognition, and chronic ischemic heart disease affects the heart's ability to pump. When these impacts happen, impairment is said to occur. Impairment does not necessarily limit functional capacity, however. The person who once used the right hand to open a jar and whose impairment prevents this might develop the strength to open it with the left hand or purchase a device to do it. Only when no alternatives remain is a disability said to result.

There are further complications to understanding disability. Definition of and determination of disability connotes difficulties in the capacity to work. In practice, however, the term is used interchangeably to connote both reduced capacity to function and the actual cessation of an activity (Yelin 1989). In the absence of compelling evidence of objective physical defect, assessment of reduced capacity to function requires that either: (1) the person report inability to perform the function, or (2) an observer reports that the person ceases the function short of full performance, including declining to undertake it. Both instances involve effort-related performance. As such, they cannot be objectively defined independently of the person's behavior. Pain-related disability, then, cannot be seen solely as a "medical" matter. Nor can it be seen as a matter of activity capacity. It is a matter of human performance, observed or reported. The purportedly disabled person performs the activity of interest, stops short of expected performance, performs it in a compromised way and with compromised effectiveness, or does not undertake the task. The criterion of performance is environmentally relational.

Defining and scaling severity of disability within the framework of the "whole person" concept has become complicated yet further by the manner in which the legal profession, abetted by health care professionals, assesses impaired performance pertaining to complex body processes. Those processes are often viewed as if they were analogous to "schedules" listing body parts impaired or missing by virtue of accident or disease, an approach based on the "whole person" concept. If performance is influenced by factors other than anatomical, physiological, or psychological processes not a part of onset, the analogy is invalidated.

DISABILITY AND LEGAL CONCEPTS

A second point is that the legal profession has accepted a test for the validity of medical advice that is compatible with an either/or view of life. Someone is either guilty or innocent, responsible for an act or not, liable or not. The test of legal responses to medical uncertainties has usually been the Draconian principle that "if something is certain to a 51% test of certainty, then it is absolutely related as cause and effect." The evolution of this perspective has a laudable objective: redress to a suffering person when events have led to a competitive performance disadvantage. However, when applied to the concepts of impairment and, from that, to disability, this perspective risks defining as a fixed characteristic of the person something that instead may be a modifiable product of the person-environment interaction. A judgment of "51% true" implies an essentially constant state when often it is not. This criterion may suffice for temporary disability status but calls into question legal perspectives on the determination of permanent disability.

Legal issues and the common law enter the discussion in another way. As Mendelson (1988) has pointed out, "In law, the tortfeasor is not entitled to complain that his victim was not a perfect specimen." How this issue is to be dealt with in allocation of indemnification in disability management is not clear. What does seem clear in light of the analysis set forth here, is that the decision to award permanent disability status should be tempered by the issues of remediability, potential beneficial effects of modifications in the environment, and of those effects dependent upon worker effort.

Disability cannot be defined independently of the actual performance of the person. A state of disability can be said to exist when the person prematurely terminates an activity, underperforms, or declines to undertake it. Disability determination may therefore be outside the scope of health care providers.

PERMANENT DISABILITY

Permanent disability status from NSLBP could not acceptably be defined solely in terms of anatomical or physiological assessments of the person, much less psychological, for the term nonspecific implies that there is no demonstrable anatomical or physiological cause. Nor could it be defined in terms of estimates of capacity to perform, for such estimates are based in significant part on behavior. Behavior, as has been shown, is inextricably bound to the environment in which it occurs. Defined in ways consonant with its behavioral aspects, disability in NSLBP should be seen as a state of activity intolerance and not a "medical" condition.

PAIN AND PSYCHOLOGICAL DISABILITY

Effects relating to nociceptive stimulation may have been at the root of the onset of a given disability state. The disability state may persist because of per-

sisting nociceptive stimulation relating to the reasons for onset, an objectively testable proposition. Disability may result from changes in the nervous system as a consequence of nociceptive stimulation that outlast the stimulation. This may occur because new sources of nociceptive stimulation arise from the early management of the problem, also objectively testable. Or, disability may occur for reasons little or not at all related to nociceptive stimulation and pain. Behavior is an essential part of the definition of disability and is related to effort and to the environment. It follows that assignment of disability status for a psychological problem, or for what is purported to be a psychological problem that arose as a consequence of a pain problem, should be seen as a psychological disability, not a pain disability. Psychiatric disorders (e.g., somatoform pain disorder, posttraumatic stress disorder) as described in DSM-IV (American Psychiatric Association 1994) can be precipitated by a work injury, and the presenting complaint by the injured person may be "pain." However these psychiatric disorders are to be defined, they should not be considered variants of "pain."

When impairment is defined within these more stringent limits, the health care system or compensation agencies should not deal with a performance problem as a pain-related permanent disability deriving from an impairment. Nor should a performance problem be considered as a pain-related permanent disability.

DISABILITY AND THE "WHOLE PERSON"

We can now return to the concept of the "whole person," an important historical root of disability programs. To the extent that a given disability involves processes that have important environmental features, the candidate for pain-related disability determination cannot be made whole without the relevant features of his/her environment also being made "whole." Disability programs based solely on making the person whole are building from a false premise when applied to human processes having environmental features. The intent of such programs is not achievable; they are pursuing a myth. The "level playing field" of opportunity to again compete in the world of work cannot be achieved without dealing with the environment. For these reasons there should be changes in the definitions of pain-related disability when applied to "effort-related" environmental conditions.

Temporary disability status can be assigned based on the report of pain and/or on observations of the person's performance or behavior. Permanent impairment based solely on complaints of NSLBP is an invalid concept. Impairment would have to be based on evidence of a nonremediable anatomical, physiological, or psychological defect. A decision in favor of permanent disability should be based not on a pain problem but, presumably, on a psychological problem. An important implication of the foregoing analysis is that, in effect, the complaint of pain in NSLBP is noncompensable in the sense of not meriting award of permanent disability status for nonspecific conditions.

TEMPORARY DISABILITY

Pain-related disabled functioning not linked exclusively to anatomical or physiological factors is in important degree a behavioral or performance phenomenon. Performance, inextricably bound to the environment as it is, cannot be seen as an "all-or-none" phenomenon. A person may be able to perform one job or set of tasks, but not another; or, perform partially but not completely. During the early phase of a back pain episode activity tolerance or the ability to perform may be totally or partially compromised (see Chapter 2) and temporary disability status may apply. At the end of an interval judged to be sufficient for healing and/or remediation, status as temporarily disabled should end. In the case of NSLBP, duration of temporary disability, if awarded, should not be assessed solely by performance of the person or by the complaint of pain.

CONSTRAINTS OF MEDICAL MANAGEMENT

In the particular case of NSLBP, constraints should be placed on applications of medical technology. The U.S. Agency for Health Care Policy and Research (AHCPR) Guidelines for back pain (Bigos et al. 1994a) and the U.K. Clinical Standards Advisory Group Report (CSAG 1994) provide an additional basis for this position (see Chapter 7). Appropriate medical care should not be denied, but rather interventions should be limited to what is consistent with temporary disability conditions and known to be effective. NSLBP is linked closely to the environment; therefore, the benefits of medical care alone are

limited. Continued treatment solely as a "medical" problem should be constrained.

SEPARATING PAIN FROM PSYCHOLOGICAL CONDITIONS

The foregoing reformulation of impairment and disability as applies to NSLBP does not address the matter of psychological factors preexisting the onset of a pain problem and exerting major influence on patient performance, or even of psychological conditions arising as an apparent consequence of persistence of a pain problem.

A person with problems of NSLBP attributed to psychological factors and with associated activity intolerance is potentially a candidate for remediation efforts as may be prescribed from appropriate evaluation. Such persons may also be candidates for temporary, or if deemed appropriate, permanent disability status with whatever benefits may accrue to those designations, though on the basis of psychological impairment, not pain.

It goes beyond the scope of this report to address in detail factors producing psychologically based disability or the remediation programs that may reduce or eliminate these factors. In line with the formulations presented above, and aside from the rarely encountered toxic, neurologically based functional defects, or frank psychoses, these conditions should be seen as embodying important environmental and effort-related features. The scope of legal and administrative disability status should be defined with due regard to these features. It is rarely, if ever, possible to make a person psychologically "whole" without consideration of the environment or milieu in which the person is to be functioning. Accordingly, a person with a psychologically based disability who enters the disability determination system with a history of adequate job performance, or in other ways having demonstrated relatively normal functioning, probably should be dealt with as temporarily disabled and having the potential for substantial remediation. Remediation may be directed to the person's psychological functioning, to modifications of the worker-job interface, or to job or career-change strategies. Dealing with such conditions in that fashion helps to diminish excessive relegation to permanent disability status and also helps maintain focus on remediation efforts.

Restricting disability status from NSLBP to temporary while psychological disability arising from it might be permanent, risks simply shifting the problem from "pain" to "psychological disability." This report advocates that psychological disability determination should be approached conceptually just as has been done with pain-related disability. To the extent that the behavior or performance of the person with so-called psychological disability is related to effort and environment, the disability should be categorized as temporary. The extent and duration of remediation efforts, or of other disability-related benefits, is an important social policy issue. However, remediation of psychological disability is a matter beyond the mandate of this report.

The responsibility of the person in effort-related matters such as these is highly germane but will be dealt with only briefly, as it is the proper subject of a detailed analysis of the conceptual bases of psychological or psychiatric disability. Clinical psychiatry and clinical psychology have for years wrestled with the question of whether mental illness and other analogous terms should be seen as forms of disease. In this context "disease" connotes some defect or functional disadvantage within the person. Reluctance to categorize a person's problem as a disease has sometimes stemmed from concerns about self-esteem or social stigma issues. Whatever may be the case, there is also the question of the effect on individual effort toward remediation. We cannot assume that patient effort can resolve or contribute greatly to resolution of psychiatric/psychological problems; though undoubtedly patient effort has an important role to play. Social and legal policy with respect to disability matters pertaining to psychiatric or psychological problems needs to be formulated with full awareness of the implications of "effort-related" matters and the effects of environmental feedback or consequences on performance.

SUMMARY

Our recommendations, if put into effect, may shift the balance between the needs of society and those of the individual. They may do so by seeming to "absolve" disability benefit programs of responsibility for performance dysfunction from nonspecific conditions. Society gains in the sense of a diminished range of responsibility; the person may lose access to previously available disability status benefits. How is that to be dealt with? As that issue relates to NSLBP, it is a question of how to redress the balance between demands of work and the person's ability to meet them. Although NSLBP does not now qualify as an impairment, it is nonetheless all too often judged as one. Our present system may arrive at permanent disability status by misusing the concept of pain and its natural course in NSLBP. Or, it may use some variant of psychological impairment as the rationale for disability assignment.

There is an alternative. Programs can and should be designed and implemented to empower the worker to gain assistance in reassessing job or career goals to ameliorate the suffering now attributed to NSLBP, but often more likely to involve work-related difficulties and the "goodness-of-fit" of worker to job (proposals are presented in Chapter 6). As with disability matters pertaining to NSLBP, the conceptual bases for disability matters relating to psychological and psychiatric problems should be carefully assessed. The needs of the individual, of employers, and of society in general, call for thorough reappraisal.

Back Pain in the Workplace: Management of Disability in Nonspecific Conditions, edited by W.E. Fordyce, IASP Press, Seattle, © 1995.

6

Prevention of Disability in the Workplace

IMPORTANCE OF THE WORKSITE

Disability status does not arise in the workplace. Injury, pain, and impairment may originate in the workplace, but disability status derives from events following an injury or the onset of the complaint of disabling pain.

Industry traditionally has looked to medicine for help in resolving the problem of work-related back pain complaints and disability. Despite the obvious advances in health care technology, the incidence and costs of disability ascribed to nonspecific low back pain (NSLBP) have continued to grow. Viewed from the perspective of the health care system, amelioration of the disability management problem, as pertains to NSLBP, has been assumed to reside mainly in establishing more effective diagnostic, therapeutic, and disability management programs within medicine. Examination of studies pertaining to what transpires in the workplace prior to an injured worker's entry into the health care delivery system suggests a rather different perspective on the problem.

In his introductory comments to the 16th Annual National Symposium on Workers' Compensation, William Hager, president of the National Council on Compensation Insurance said, "Unless we get unneeded services and providers out of the workers' compensation system, the house will come down" (Hager 1993). Frymoyer and Cats-Baril (1991) have raised the question: "Have medical professionals of all types become part of the problem, rather than part of the solution?"

Worksite-based programs intended both to prevent back injuries and to facilitate return to work without recourse to medical intervention have received increasing attention. Results from these programs suggest that a major portion of the NSLBP disability problem may be subject to amelioration *before* the health care delivery system becomes involved. Effectiveness of interventions for reduction of dis-

ability that bear little if any relationship to anatomical or neurophysiological issues lends further support to this approach. We must question the extent to which complaints of back pain in NSLBP are "medical" problems for a significant number of those who become care-seekers.

EMPLOYER POLICIES

Rousmaniere (1990) has claimed that approximately 50% of costs resulting from workplace injuries depends on how the company manages injuries after they occur. Habeck et al. (1991) reported confirming data when they found that firms performing disability management methods poorly, when compared with companies using effective methods, had twice as many recordable injury events but four times as many workers' compensation claims. Thus, rate of subsequent disability assignment was more effective than rate of injuries in distinguishing effective from ineffective employer policies.

Robertson and Keeve (1983) studied worksite efforts to prevent industrial back injury claims by minimizing physical hazards through developing and enforcing safety and health regulations. They reported a significant decrease in objectively verifiable injuries such as lacerations and fractures. However, more subjective injury complaints such as back "strains" were unaffected. "Objectively verifiable" injuries, as applied to back pain, are interpreted to relate to "specific back pain" and subjective injuries to NSLBP. Undoubtedly safety and ergonomic factors contribute to the incidence of back injury. However, their relationship to care-seeking for NSLBP is much less evident.

Waddell (1994) recently carried out an exhaustive review of the international literature on epidemiology of back pain. In synthesizing the data bearing on physical demands of work, he said: "There is general

37

though not unanimous agreement that back pain and probably also degenerative changes in the spine are more common in people in heavy manual occupations and undertaking heavy lifting. . . . The balance of the evidence is that it is the duration rather than the frequency of spells off work with back pain that is increased in those with heavy physical work."

Hunt and Habeck (1993) studied the relationship of three sets of employer policy and practice methods with disability outcome measures pertaining to all injuries or diseases, not just back pain. They studied 220 Michigan companies of 100 or more employees distributed among seven industries. The first policy or practice domain studied was safety intervention designed to prevent injuries from occurring. The second was disability management designed to minimize the disability consequences of a given injury, for example, case monitoring and proactive return to work. The third was health promotion: attempts to intervene with the individual worker to encourage more healthy life-styles in the expectation that this might reduce lost work time. Another set of corporate culture measures was applied to assess the general attitude and practice of the firm toward disability management or reduction procedures.

Results indicated that employer diligence on matters of work safety was strongly associated with better disability outcomes, as were policies providing for proactive return-to-work programs. They state: "The twin strategies of trying to prevent injuries in the first place, and working to ameliorate their disability effects through disability management techniques, are both shown to be productive in reducing workplace disability in those establishments that have implemented them rigorously." Diligent safety programs improved performance by reducing lost workdays by 13.0%; systematic safety training programs reduced them by 6.53%. Ergonomic solutions, however, resulted in no reduction in lost workdays. Similarly, emphasis on systematic return-to-work programs reduced lost workdays by 13.59% but reliance on case monitoring and wellness orientation did not (under those approaches, lost workdays in fact increased by 10.18% and 1.61%, respectively) (Hunt and Habeck 1993).

Failure of this study to find "wellness enhancing" programs effective in reducing disability rates has several possible interpretations. One is that those programs did not have a sufficiently beneficial effect on worker health or wellness. The study design did not

permit analysis of that factor. A second possible reason for failure of wellness programs to reduce disability must be considered. A worker's self-perception as disabled and requiring medical intervention may not be related to "wellness" in a general sense. Perception as disabled may, instead, be related to mood or to various cognitive perceptions about the meaning of extant body sensations somewhat irrespective of more general perceptions of "wellness."

The failure of focus on ergonomic factors to influence disability outcome does not establish that ergonomic factors are unimportant. But, as has been shown, complaints of pain, subsequent care-seeking, and probability of eventual assignment to long-term disability status, are not randomly distributed in the worker population. They occur more in some segments of the population than others. The limited relationship between heavy work and disability award for NSLBP, and the failure of ergonomic emphasis to markedly reduce disability rates, suggests that more is involved than physical demands of the job. The relative contribution of ergonomic factors to a given job or job injury probably varies from one situation to another.

Companies that choose to focus on ergonomic factors may also, thereby, fail to emphasize disability management strategies. The Hunt and Habeck findings suggest that disability management may exert even more influence on care-seeking behavior. Effects of the policies and procedures studied as applied only to NSLBP cannot be assessed directly from the Hunt and Habeck study. However, there are two sources from which inferences about the comparability of low back pain to other conditions can be drawn. Data from the Boeing study suggest that predictors of illness-related absenteeism for low back pain are essentially the same as for other conditions reported (Battié et al. 1993; Bigos et al. 1992). That observation suggests that whatever factors influence persistence of disability may have a significant level of comparability for other conditions. The second source is derived logically from the analysis carried out in Chapter 3 regarding ambiguities in pain and suffering and their apparent impact on incidence and persistence of NSLBP complaints and the studies from which that analysis drew. That analysis implies that many workers entering the health care system with complaints of back pain found to be nonspecific are being influenced by factors beyond the domain of pain and nociception, per se.

PROACTIVE PREVENTION POLICY

The major focus of the Task Force on Pain in the Workplace is on NSLBP and its relation to health care. A major analysis of worksite interventions to prevent disability goes beyond the emphasis and the collective expertise of task force. Nonetheless, worksite-based interventions for preventing long-term disability from NSLBP are important matters. They will receive some, albeit limited, consideration in this report.

Prevailing work injury management strategies operate from a health care provider-based framework. It is a reactive approach. Habeck (1993) comments, "As work disability increases, providers expand efforts to offer more and better rehabilitation services; however, due to the reactive nature of this model these efforts fail to address the underlying causes of the problem. As a result, many providers continue to function from a 'broken paradigm' that can only offer limited solutions to work disability and may actually contribute to escalating costs of health care and rehabilitation in disability benefit programs. The consequences of this broken paradigm are felt not only by payers and recipients of the system but are genuinely harmful to the viability of service providers." That broken paradigm fails to adequately differentiate pain from suffering and thereby treats suffering as if it were pain.

An alternative to the reactive approach is to recognize the potential of workplace disability prevention programs to reduce health care costs and the incidence of long-term disability. This proactive approach seeks to prevent primary occurrence of injuries, for example, through work safety programs. It seeks to facilitate return to work as an active part of medical management, should that referral occur. However, it also seeks to influence worker readiness to continue on the job rather than prematurely or inappropriately seeking medical care.

Owens (1993) comments: "Disability management reflects the employer's overall human resource philosophy. Employers who need skilled workers for complex jobs and place a high value on the people who work for them will provide more in benefits to attract and retain their employees. In such an environment, disability management is aimed at preventing disability and, when it inevitably occurs, providing accommodation and adequate compensation to replace lost wages while encouraging rehabilitation and return to work."

Habeck (1993) summarizes proactive employer or worksite-based objectives for disability prevention and management as:

- Prevent occurrence of accidents and disability.

- Intervene early for disability risk factors.

- Coordinate services for cost-effective restoration and return to work.

Habeck (1993) has formulated more detailed recommendations for employer strategies for effective disability management:

1. Recognize signs and symptoms of worker impairment.

2. Develop *early* interventions and *preventive* responses to potential work disruptions.

3. Monitor injured/disabled workers *responsively.*

4. Identify, utilize, and evaluate *qualified* health care and occupational medicine providers.

5. Influence *employee selection* of treatment and rehabilitation services.

6. Create labor/management agreements that facilitate work return and worker retention planning.

7. Promote disability management policies and procedures and corresponding protocols for case management.

8. Generate *light duty options* and realistic work return transition opportunities for impaired workers.

9. Accommodate injured/disabled workers by *job site redesigns and modifications.*

10. Implement *health promotion and wellness programs* for stress management, alcohol and substance abuse, weight control, hypertension reduction, and smoking cessation.

It is beyond the scope of this report to develop in further detail the empirical and conceptual basis for workplace-based changes in management of injury and disability and procedural details for their implementation. Detailed discussions of the issues involved and of remediation strategies can be found in Boschen (1992), Galvin (1992), Owens (1993), and Roessler (1988).

It should be evident that worksite interventions are powerful and essential forces for managing and preventing disability from NSLBP. Those ameliorating effects have addressed disability and worker decisions to continue or discontinue work. They have not in any direct sense addressed "pain" except in the sense of seeking to prevent accidents from which "pain" may derive. However, as was pointed out in the previous discussion and review of data bearing on worker decisions to seek help for pain, the conceptualization of pain and its relationship to impairment and disability points clearly to the importance of recognizing that chronic NSLBP is far more than a medical problem. It has medical features. But it also has many features linked intimately to worksite and other environmental factors.

Worksite factors, including the kinds of company policies studied by Hunt and Habeck (1993), and as described in the review by Battié (1992), seem clearly to be playing major roles in disability outcomes. The positive effects of these factors, occurring before advent of medical care, cast further doubts upon the validity of medically based definitions of NSLBP. As has been discussed in Chapter 3, a significant part of the problem of disability related to NSLBP is the unneeded medicalization of what is in significant degree a problem of more generalized suffering; suffering that may be only tangentially—if at all—related to anatomical or physiological factors in the low back.

IMPLICATIONS FOR EMPLOYERS

The positive effects on productivity and company objectives from enhanced worker identification with and participation in job performance needs no reiteration here. However, the influence of these factors on care-seeking and the seeking or acceptance of disability status has not been well recognized.

One implication of this report for employers is that reductions in disability rates with the associated costs and losses of productivity may be achieved by increasing emphasis on enhancing the social and psychological milieu of the worksite. Pain and inability to continue work are complex personal perceptions and judgments. They are influenced by the social and psychological milieu of the worksite. The more that the worker has a positive identification with job performance and relations with co-workers, the greater the likelihood that personal distress will intrude less into performance. If that distress is related to transitory body discomfort, the more likely the worker will rely

on the natural healing course and continued job participation rather than seeking medically sanctioned time out from work. This is not to suggest that a worker should persist in job effort irrespective of experienced pain. The point is that how well a person feels and anticipations of future consequences based on body sensations are related to the work environment. Strengthening the bond between worker and worksite can have a positive effect on care-seeking and on readiness to persist in assigned disability status.

A second implication of this report for employers is the importance of recognizing that health care professionals often view pain problems somewhat exclusively from the perspective of a disease model with the resultant tendency to confound pain with suffering and specificity with nonspecificity. They thereby encourage excessive time of reduced activity levels and inappropriate assignment of disability status. Disability management procedures established by employers can track the medical management of injured workers and facilitate timely return to work. This issue is discussed further in Chapters 8 and 9.

A third implication for employers is that worksite-based efforts to enhance identification with the job may be a more powerful way of containing disability costs than are pre-employment screening programs. Those aspects of screening focused on avoiding losses or costs associated with future disability are based on the assumption that psychological and other intrapersonal factors purported to be measured by pre-employment screening are major forces in determining future job performance, including avoiding persisting disability. Obvious psychological and intrapersonal difficulty issues are presumably already a factor in personnel selection. However, the findings on which this report draws suggest that, with respect to NSLBP and several other nonspecific conditions, rate and persistence of disability may be influenced more by worksite factors. Pre-employment screening is unlikely to be an adequate substitute for worksite enhancement as a method for reducing disability costs for NSLBP. It also violates concepts of a level playing field

ACTIVITY INTOLERANCE AND JOB FLEXIBILITY

There are many reasons for activity intolerance. One is pain. Another is more generalized suffering.

People who suffer often use the language of pain to describe their feelings (Loeser 1980). Because language is a reflection of and constraint upon thought, we should not be surprised that they ascribe their suffering to a specific injury that they believe is the cause of their pain and, thence, suffering. It is through this linkage that suffering, from any cause, may lead to activity intolerance ascribed to NSLBP. A third reason for activity intolerance is limitation from physiological or anatomical factors.

Suffering may develop in response to long-standing and unresolved pain problems or as an expression of emotional distress. That distress may relate to emotional problems unrelated to work or it may arise as a consequence of job-worker interaction. Work-related suffering may arise because the job requires skills, speed of performance, precision of performance, strength and endurance, or, in some other manner, coping skills greater than the worker can provide. The job may have been a poor fit with worker abilities from the outset or it may have evolved into one. Changes in the worker as a result of injury, aging, or for some other reason may make a previously adequate job-worker fit no longer tenable. Those and other possible reasons may underlie worker distress, suffering, and activity intolerance in relation to a job.

The particular reasons for activity intolerance are less important than the question of whether the condition is remediable. Remedy might come from changes in the job, changes in the worker from skill or stress management training, etc., or by a change to work providing a better fit. It also can come from restoration of function through healing of the injury or through a reformulation of the meaning of painful stimuli.

Back Pain in the Workplace: Management of Disability in Nonspecific Conditions, edited by W.E. Fordyce, IASP Press, Seattle, © 1995.

7

Early Management of Nonspecific Low Back Pain

This chapter addresses medical management of the recent onset back pain problem diagnosed as nonspecific. The U.S. Agency for Health Care Policy and Research (AHCPR) was mandated by Congress to develop clinically relevant guidelines for health care providers and consumers on a variety of important health problems. One of those was low back pain (Bigos et al. 1994a). The panel of experts brought together to develop low back pain guidelines included representatives from several countries. Several members of that panel also are members or consultants to the Task Force on Pain in the Workplace. It was the decision of the task force, and with the generous permission of AHCPR, to use appropriate selections from those low back pain guidelines for this chapter. A similar report has been prepared for the United Kingdom by the Clinical Standards Advisory Group (CSAG 1994). Selected elements of that report are also reproduced below by permission.

We include these excerpts because we believe that concepts currently used for the medical management of the complaint of low back pain are major contributors to the epidemic of disability ascribed to nonspecific low back pain (NSLBP). The expert panels that created these reports do not need duplication for this report, as everything that needs to be said is contained within these documents. Those who wish to provide solutions to the problems of NSLBP and its associated disability must address not only workplace factors but also the often misguided health care that increases the risk of disability. Documents on this subject originated in both the United Kingdom and the United States and indicate the widespread recognition that changing health care for NSLBP is an essential step in addressing the epidemic of disability ascribed to NSLBP.

EXCERPTS FROM
ACUTE LOW BACK PROBLEMS IN ADULTS: ASSESSMENT AND TREATMENT
by S. Bigos (panel chair) et al., Quick Reference Guide for Clinicians, AHCPR Publication no. 95-0643, U.S. Department of Health and Human Services, Public Health Service, Agency for Health Care Policy and Research, Rockville, Md., 1994b

PURPOSE AND SCOPE

Low back problems affect virtually everyone at some time during their life. Surveys indicate a yearly prevalence of symptoms in 50% of working age adults; 15–20% seek medical care. Low back problems rank high among the reasons for physician office visits and are costly in terms of medical treatment, lost productivity, and nonmonetary costs such as diminished ability to perform or enjoy usual activities. In fact, for persons under age 45, low back problems

are the most common cause of disability.

Acute low back problems are defined as activity intolerance due to lower back or back-related leg symptoms of less than three months' duration. About 90% of patients with acute low back problems spontaneously recover activity tolerance within one month. The approach to a new episode in a patient with a recurrent low back problem is similar to that of a new acute episode.

The findings and recommendations included in the *Clinical Practice Guideline* define a paradigm shift away from focusing care exclusively on the pain and toward helping patients improve activity tolerance. The intent of this *Quick Reference Guide* is to bring to life this paradigm shift. The guide provides information on the detection of serious conditions that occasionally cause low back symptoms (conditions such as spinal fracture, tumor, infection, cauda equina syndrome, or nonspinal conditions). However, treatment of these conditions is beyond the scope of this guideline. In addition, the guideline does not address the care of patients younger than 18 years or those with chronic back problems (back-related activity limitations of greater than three months' duration).

INITIAL ASSESSMENT

- Seek potentially dangerous underlying conditions.

- In the absence of signs of dangerous conditions, there is no need for special studies since 90% of patients will recover spontaneously within four weeks.

A focused medical history and physical examination are sufficient to assess the patient with an acute or recurrent limitation due to low back symptoms of less than four weeks' duration. Patient responses and findings on the history and physical examination, referred to as "red flags" (Table 6), raise suspicion of serious underlying spinal conditions. Their absence rules out the need for special studies during the first four weeks of symptoms when spontaneous recovery is expected. The medical history and physical examination can also alert the clinician to nonspinal pathology (abdominal, pelvic, thoracic) that can present as low back symptoms. Acute low back symptoms can then be classified into one of three working categories:

- *Potentially serious spinal condition*—tumor, infection, spinal fracture, or a major neurologic compromise, such as cauda equina syndrome, suggested by a red flag.

- *Sciatica*—back-related lower limb symptoms suggesting lumbosacral nerve root compromise.

- *Nonspecific back symptoms*—occurring primarily in the back and suggesting neither nerve root compromise nor a serious underlying condition.

MEDICAL HISTORY

In addition to detecting serious conditions and categorizing back symptoms, the medical history es-

Table 6
Red flags for potentially serious conditions

Possible Fracture	Possible Tumor or Infection	Possible Cauda Equina Syndrome
From medical history		
Major trauma, such as vehicle accident or fall from height Minor trauma or even strenuous lifting (in older and potentially osteoporotic patient)	Age over 50 or under 20 History of cancer Constitutional symptoms, such as recent fever or chills or unexplained weight loss Risk factors for spinal infection: recent bacterial infection (e.g., urinary tract infection); IV drug abuse; or immune suppression (from steroids, transplant, or HIV) Pain that worsens when supine; severe nighttime pain	Saddle anesthesia Recent onset of bladder dysfunction, such as urinary retention, increased frequency, or overflow incontinence Severe or progressive neurologic deficit in the lower extremity
From physical examination		
		Unexpected laxity of the anal sphincter Perianal/perineal sensory loss Major motor weakness: quadriceps (knee extension weakness); ankle plantar flexors, evertors, and dorsiflexors (foot drop)

tablishes rapport between the clinician and patient. The patient's description of present symptoms and limitations, duration of symptoms, and history of previous episodes defines the problem. It also provides insight into concerns, expectations, and non-physical (psychological and socioeconomic) issues that may alter the patient's response to treatment. Assessment tools such as pain drawings and visual analog pain-rating scales may help further document the patient's perceptions and progress.

A patient's estimate of personal activity intolerance due to low back symptoms contributes to the clinical assessment of the severity of the back problem, guides treatment, and establishes a baseline for recommending daily activities and evaluating progress.

Open-ended questions, such as those listed below, can gauge the need for further discussion or specific inquiries for more detailed information:

- *What are your symptoms?*
  Pain, numbness, weakness, stiffness?
  Located primarily in back, leg, or both?
  Constant or intermittent?

- *How do these symptoms limit you?*
  How long can you sit, stand, walk?
  How much weight can you lift?

- *When did the current limitations begin?*
  How long have your activities been limited?
  More than four weeks?
  Have you had similar episodes previously?
  Previous testing or treatment?

- *What do you hope we can accomplish during this visit?*

PHYSICAL EXAMINATION

The examination is mostly subjective since patient response or interpretation is required for all parts except reflex testing and circumferential measurements for atrophy.

Addressing red flags

Physical examination evidence of severe neurologic compromise that correlates with the medical history may indicate a need for immediate consultation. The examination may further modify suspicions of tumor, infection, or significant trauma. A medical history suggestive of nonspinal pathology mimicking a back problem may warrant examination of pulses, abdomen, pelvis, or other areas.

Observation and regional back examination

Limping or coordination problems indicate the need for specific neurologic testing. Severe guarding of lumbar motion in all planes may support a suspected diagnosis of spinal infection, tumor, or fracture. However, given marked variations among persons with and without symptoms, range-of-motion measurements of the back are of limited value.

Vertebral point tenderness to palpation, when associated with other signs or symptoms, may be suggestive of but not specific for spinal fracture or infection. Palpable soft-tissue tenderness is, by itself, an even less specific or reliable finding.

Neurologic screening

The neurologic examination can focus on a few tests that seek evidence of nerve root impairment, peripheral neuropathy, or spinal cord dysfunction. Over 90% of all clinically significant lower extremity radiculopathy due to disc herniation involves the L5 or S1 nerve root at the L4-5 or L5-S1 disc level.

- *Testing for Muscle Strength.* The patient's inability to toe walk (calf muscles, mostly S1 nerve root), heel walk (ankle and toe dorsiflexor muscles, L5 and some L4 nerve roots), or do a single squat and rise (quadriceps muscles, mostly L4 nerve root) may indicate muscle weakness. Specific testing of the dorsiflexor muscles of the ankle or great toe (suggestive of L5 or some L4 nerve root dysfunction), hamstrings and ankle evertors (L5-S1), and toe flexors (S1) is also important.

- *Circumferential Measurements.* Muscle atrophy can be detected by circumferential measurements of the calf and thigh bilaterally. Differences of less than 2 cm in measurements of the two limbs at the same level may be a normal variation. Symmetrical muscle bulk and strength are expected unless the patient has a neurologic impairment or a history of lower extremity muscle or joint problem.

- *Reflexes.* The ankle jerk reflex tests mostly the S1 nerve root and the knee jerk reflex tests mostly the L4 nerve root; neither tests the L5 nerve root. The reliability of reflex testing can be diminished

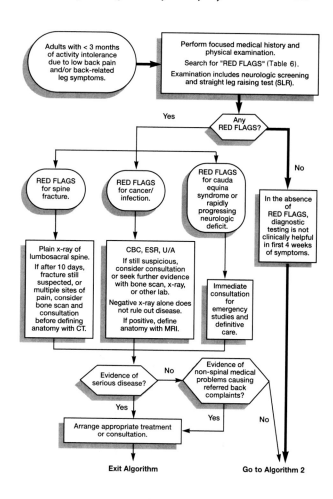

Algorithm 1. Initial evaluation of acute low back problem.

in the presence of adjacent joint or muscle problems. Up-going toes in response to stroking the plantar footpad (Babinski or plantar response) may indicate upper motor-neuron abnormalities (such as myelopathy or demyelinating disease) rather than a common low back problem.

- *Sensory Examination.* Testing light touch or pressure in the medial (L4), dorsal (L5), and lateral (S1) aspects of the foot is usually sufficient for sensory screening.

Clinical tests for sciatic tension

The straight leg raising (SLR) test can detect tension on the L5 and/or S1 nerve root. SLR may reproduce leg pain by stretching nerve roots irritated by a disc herniation.

Pain below the knee at less than 70 degrees of straight leg raising, aggravated by dorsiflexion of the ankle and relieved by ankle plantar flexion or external

limb rotation, is most suggestive of tension on the L5 or S1 nerve root related to disc herniation. Reproducing back pain alone with SLR testing does not indicate significant nerve root tension.

Crossover pain occurs when straight raising of the patient's well limb elicits pain in the leg with sciatica. Crossover pain is a stronger indication of nerve root compression than pain elicited from raising the straight painful limb.

Sitting knee extension can also test sciatic tension. The patient with significant nerve root irritation tends to complain or lean backward to reduce tension on the nerve.

INCONSISTENT FINDINGS AND PAIN BEHAVIOR

The patient who embellishes a medical history, exaggerates pain drawings, or provides responses on physical examination inconsistent with known physiology can be particularly challenging. A strongly positive supine straight leg raising test without complaint on sitting knee extension and inconsistent responses on examination raise a suspicion that non-physical factors may be affecting the patient's responses. "Pain behaviors" (verbal or nonverbal communication of distress or suffering) such as amplified grimacing, distorted gait or posture, moaning, and rubbing of painful body parts may also cloud medical issues and even evoke angry responses from the clinician.

Interpreting inconsistencies or pain behaviors as malingering does not benefit the patient or the clinician. It is more useful to view such behavior and inconsistencies as the patient's attempt to enlist the practitioner as an advocate, a plea for help. The patient could be trapped in a job where activity requirements are unrealistic relative to the person's age or health. In some cases, the patient may be negotiating with an insurer or be involved in legal actions. In patients with recurrent back problems, inconsistencies and amplifications may simply be habits learned during previous medical evaluations. In working with these patients, the clinician should attempt to identify any psychological or socioeconomic pressures that might be influenced in a positive manner. The overall goal should always be to facilitate the patient's recovery and avoid the development of chronic low back disability.

INITIAL CARE

PATIENT EDUCATION

If the initial assessment detects no serious condition, assure the patient that there is "no hint of a dangerous problem" and that "a rapid recovery can be expected." The need for education will vary among patients and during various stages of care. An obviously apprehensive patient may require a more detailed explanation. Patients with sciatica may have a longer expected recovery time than patients with nonspecific back symptoms and thus may need more education and reassurance. Any patient who does not recover within a few weeks may need more extensive education about back problems and the reassurance that special studies may be considered if recovery is slow.

PATIENT COMFORT

Comfort is often a patient's first concern. Nonprescription analgesics will provide sufficient pain relief for most patients with acute low back symptoms. If treatment response is inadequate, as evidenced by continued symptoms and activity limitations, prescribed pharmaceuticals or physical methods may be added. Comorbid conditions, side effects, cost, and provider/patient preference should guide the clinician's choice of recommendations. Table 7 summarizes comfort options.

Oral pharmaceuticals

The safest effective medication for acute low back problems appears to be acetaminophen. Nonsteroidal anti-inflammatory drugs (NSAIDs), including aspirin and ibuprofen, are also effective although they can cause gastrointestinal irritation/ulceration or (less commonly) renal or allergic problems. Phenyl-

Table 7
Symptom control methods

Recommended		
Nonprescription analgesics		
Acetaminophen (safest) NSAIDs (Aspirin,[1] ibuprofen[1])		
Prescribed pharmaceutical methods	**Prescribed physical methods**	
Nonspecific low back symptoms and/or sciatica	*Nonspecific low back symptoms*	*Sciatica*
Other NSAIDs[1]	Manipulation (in place of medication or a shorter trial if combined with NSAIDs)	
Options		
Nonspecific low back symptoms and/or sciatica	*Nonspecific low back symptoms*	*Sciatica*
Muscle relaxants[2,3,4] Opioids[2,3,4]	Physical agents and modalities[2] (heat or cold modalities for home programs only) Shoe insoles[2]	Manipulation (in place of medication or a shorter trial if combined with NSAIDs) Physical agents and modalities[2] (heat or cold modalities for home programs only) Few days' rest[4] Shoe insoles[2]

[1] Aspirin and other NSAIDs are not recommended for use in combination with one another due to the risk of GI complications.
[2] Equivocal efficacy.
[3] Significant potential for producing drowsiness and debilitation; potential for dependency.
[4] Short course (few days only) for severe symptoms.

Initial visit

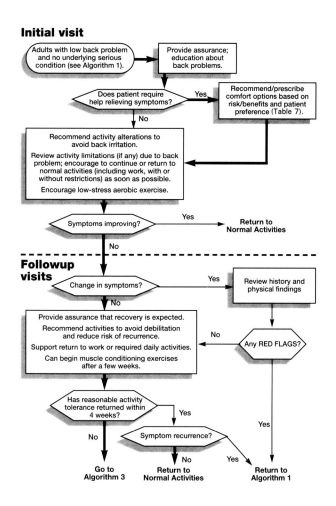

Algorithm 2. Treatment of acute low back problem on initial and followup visits.

butazone is not recommended due to risks of bone marrow suppression. Acetaminophen may be used safely in combination with NSAIDs or other pharmacologic or physical therapeutics, especially in otherwise healthy patients.

Muscle relaxants seem no more effective than NSAIDs for treating patients with low back symptoms, and using them in combination with NSAIDs has no demonstrated benefit. Side effects including drowsiness have been reported in up to 30% of patients taking muscle relaxants.

Opioids appear no more effective than safer analgesics for managing low back symptoms. Opioids should be avoided if possible and, when chosen, used only for a short time. Poor patient tolerance and risks of drowsiness, decreased reaction time, clouded judgment, and potential misuse/dependence have been reported in up to 35% of patients. Patients should be warned of these potentially debilitating problems

Physical methods

- *Manipulation,* defined as manual loading of the spine using short or long leverage methods, is safe and effective for patients in the first month a of acute low back symptoms without radiculopathy. For patients with symptoms lasting longer than one month, manipulation is probably safe but its efficacy is unproven. If manipulation has not resulted in symptomatic and functional improvement after four weeks, it should be stopped and the patient reevaluated.

- *Traction* applied to the spine has not been found effective for treating acute low back symptoms.

- *Physical modalities* such as *massage, diathermy, ultrasound, cutaneous laser treatment, biofeedback, and transcutaneous electrical nerve stimulation (TENS)* also have no proven efficacy in the treatment of acute low back symptoms. If requested, the clinician may wish to provide the patient with instructions on self-application of heat or cold therapy for temporary symptom relief.

- *Invasive techniques* such as *needle acupuncture* and *injection procedures* (injection of trigger points in the back; injection of facet joints; injection of steroids, lidocaine, or opioids in the epidural space) have no proven benefit in the treatment of acute low back symptoms.

- *Other miscellaneous therapies* have been evaluated. No evidence indicates that *shoe lifts* are effective in treating acute low back symptoms or limitations, especially when the difference in lower limb length is less than 2 cm. Shoe insoles are a safe and inexpensive option if requested by patients with low back symptoms who must stand for prolnged periods. Low back corsets and back belts, however, do not appear beneficial for treating acute low back symptoms.

ACTIVITY ALTERATION

To avoid both undue back irritation and debilitation from inactivity, recommendations for alternate activity can be helpful. Most patients will not require bed rest. Prolonged bed rest (more than four days) has potential debilitating effects, and its efficacy in the treatment of acute low back problems is unproven. Two to four days of bed rest are reserved for patients with the most severe limitations (due primarily to leg pain).

Avoiding undue back irritation

Activities and postures that increase stress on the back also tend to aggravate back symptoms. Patients limited by back symptoms can minimize the stress of lifting by keeping any lifted object close to the body at the level of the navel. Twisting, bending, and reaching while lifting also increase stress on the back. Sitting, although safe, may aggravate symptoms for some patients. Advise these patients to avoid prolonged sitting and to change position often. A soft support placed at the small of the back, armrests to support some body weight, and a slight recline of the chair back may make required sitting more comfortable.

Avoiding debilitation

Until the patient returns to normal activity, aerobic (endurance) conditioning exercise such as walking, stationary biking, swimming, and even light jogging may be recommended to help avoid debilitation from inactivity. An incremental, gradually increasing regimen of aerobic exercise (up to 20 to 30 minutes daily) can usually be started within the first two weeks of symptoms. Such conditioning activities have been found to stress the back no more than sitting for an equal time period on the side of the bed. Patients should be informed that exercise may increase symptoms slightly at first. If intolerable, some exercise alteration is usually helpful.

Conditioning exercises for trunk muscles are more mechanically stressful to the back than aerobic exercise. Such exercises are not recommended during the first few weeks of symptoms, although they may later help patients regain and maintain activity tolerance.

There is no evidence to indicate that back-specific exercise machines are effective for treating acute low back problems. Neither is there evidence that stretching of the back helps patients with acute symptoms.

Work activities

When requested, clinicians may choose to offer specific instructions about activity at work for patients with acute limitations due to low back symptoms. The patient's age, general health, and perceptions of safe limits of sitting, standing, walking, or lifting (noted on initial history) can help provide reasonable starting points for activity recommendations. The clinician should make clear to patients and employers that:

- Even moderately heavy unassisted lifting may aggravate back symptoms.

- Any restrictions are intended to allow for spontaneous recovery or time to build activity tolerance through exercise.

Activity restrictions are prescribed for a short time period only, depending upon work requirements (no benefits apparent beyond three months).

SPECIAL STUDIES AND DIAGNOSTIC CONSIDERATIONS

Routine testing (laboratory tests, plain x-rays of the lumbosacral spine) and imaging studies are not recommended during the first month of activity limitation due to back symptoms except when a red flag noted on history or examination raises suspicion of a dangerous low back or nonspinal condition. If a patient's limitations due to low back symptoms do not improve in four weeks, reassessment is recommended. After again reviewing the patient's activity limitations, history, and physical findings, the clinician may then consider further diagnostic studies, and discuss these with the patient.

TIMING AND LIMITS OF SPECIAL STUDIES

Waiting four weeks before considering special tests allows 90% of patients to recover spontaneously and avoids unneeded procedures. This also reduces the potential confusion of falsely labeling age-related changes on imaging studies (commonly noted in patients older than 30 without back symptoms) as the cause of the acute symptoms. In the absence of either red flags or persistent activity limitations due to continuous limb symptoms, imaging studies (especially plain x-rays) rarely provide information that changes the clinical approach to the acute low back problem.

SELECTION OF SPECIAL STUDIES

Prior to ordering imaging studies the clinician should have noted either of the following:

- The emergence of a red flag.

- Physiologic evidence of tissue insult or neurologic dysfunction.

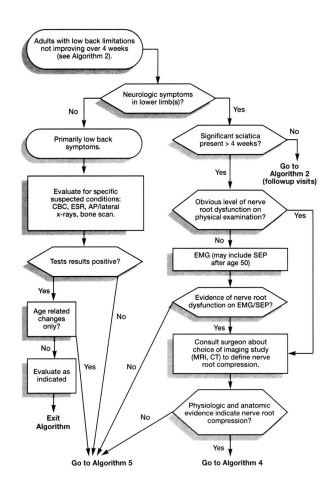

Algorithm 3. Evaluation of the slow-to-recover patient (symptoms > 4 weeks).

Physiologic evidence may be in the form of definitive nerve findings on physical examination, electrodiagnostic studies (when evaluating sciatica), and a laboratory test or bone scan (when evaluating nonspecific low back symptoms). Unquestionable findings that identify specific nerve root compromise on the neurologic examination are sufficient physiologic evidence to warrant imaging. When the neurologic examination is less clear, however, further physiologic evidence of nerve root dysfunction should be considered before ordering an imaging study. Electromyography (EMG) including H-reflex tests may be useful to identify subtle focal neurologic dysfunction in patients with leg symptoms lasting longer than three to four weeks. Sensory evoked potentials (SEPs) may be added to the assessment if spinal stenosis or spinal cord myelopathy is suspected.

Laboratory tests such as erythrocyte sedimentation rate (ESR), complete blood count (CBC), and urinalysis (UA) can be useful to screen for nonspecific medical diseases (especially infection and tumor) of the low back. A bone scan can detect physiologic reactions to suspected spinal tumor, infection, or occult fracture.

Should physiologic evidence indicate tissue insult or nerve impairment, discuss with a consultant selection of an imaging test to define a potential anatomic cause (CT for bone, MRI for neural or other soft tissue). Anatomic definition is commonly needed to guide surgery or specific procedures. Selection of an imaging test should also take into consideration any patient allergies to contrast media (myelogram) or concerns about claustrophobia (MRI) and costs. A discussion with a specialist on selection of the most clinically valuable study can often assist the primary care clinician to avoid duplication. Table 8 provides a general comparison of the abilities of different techniques to identify physiologic insult and define anatomic defects. Missing from the table is discography, which is not recommended for assessing patients with acute low back symptoms.

Table 8
Ability of different techniques to identify
and define pathology

Technique	Identify Physiologic Insult	Define Anatomic Defect
History	+	+
Physical examination:		
Circumference measurements	+	+
Reflexes	++	++
Straight leg raising (SLR)	++	+
Crossed SLR	+++	++
Motor	++	++
Sensory	++	++
Laboratory studies (ESR, CBC, UA)	++	0
Bone scan[1]	+++	++
EMG/SEP	+++	++
X-ray[1]	0	+
CT[1]	0	++++[2]
MRI	0	++++[2]
Myelo-CT[1]	0	++++[2]
Myelography[1]	0	++++[2]

Note: Number of plus signs indicates relative ability to identify or define.
[1]Risk of complications (radiation, infection, etc.): highest for myelo-CT, second highest for myelography, and relatively less risk for bone scan, x-ray, and CT.
[2]False-positive diagnostic findings in up to 30% of people without symptoms at age 30.

In general, an imaging study may be an appropriate consideration for the patient whose limitations due to consistent symptoms have persisted for one month or more:

- When surgery is being considered for treatment of a specific detectable loss of neurologic function.

- To further evaluate potentially serious spinal pathology.

Reliance upon imaging studies alone to evaluate the source of low back symptoms, however, carries a significant risk of diagnostic confusion, given the possibility of falsely identifying a finding that was present before symptoms began.

MANAGEMENT CONSIDERATIONS AFTER SPECIAL STUDIES

Definitive treatment for serious conditions (see Table 6) detected by special studies is beyond the scope of this guideline. When special studies fail to define the exact cause of symptoms, however, no patient should receive an impression that the clinician thinks "nothing is wrong" or that the problem could be "in their head." Assure the patient that a clinical workup is highly successful in detecting serious conditions, but does not reveal the precise cause of most low back symptoms.

SURGICAL CONSIDERATIONS

Within the first three months of acute low back symptoms, surgery is considered only when serious spinal pathology or nerve root dysfunction obviously due to a herniated lumbar disc is detected. A disc herniation, characterized by protrusion of the central nucleus pulposus through a defect in the outer annulus fibrosis, may trap a nerve root causing irritation, leg symptoms, and nerve root dysfunction. The presence of a herniated lumbar disc on an imaging study, however, does not necessarily imply nerve root dysfunction. Studies of asymptomatic adults commonly demonstrate intervertebral disc herniations that apparently do not entrap a nerve root or cause symptoms.

Therefore, nerve root decompression can be considered for a patient if all of the following criteria exist:

- Sciatica is both severe and disabling.

- Symptoms of sciatica persist without improvement for longer than four weeks or with extreme progression.

- There is strong physiologic evidence of dysfunction of a specific nerve root with intervertebral disc herniation confirmed at the corresponding level and side by findings on an imaging study.

Patients with acute low back pain alone, without findings of serious conditions or significant nerve root compression, rarely benefit from a surgical consultation.

Many patients with strong clinical findings of nerve root dysfunction due to disc herniation recover activity tolerance within one month; no evidence indicates that delaying surgery for this period worsens outcomes. With or without an operation, more than 80% of patients with obvious surgical indications eventually recover. Surgery seems to be a luxury for speeding recovery of patients with obvious surgical indications but benefits fewer than 40% of patients

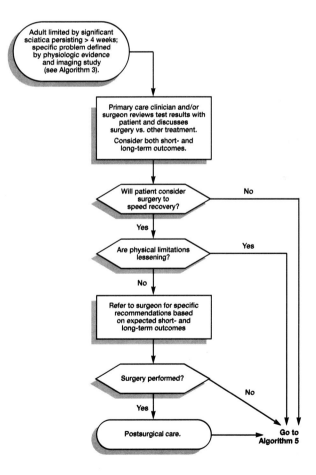

Algorithm 4. Surgical considerations for patients with persistent sciatica.

with questionable physiologic findings. Moreover, surgery increases the chance of future procedures with higher complication rates. Overall, the incidence of first-time disc surgery complications, including infection and bleeding, is less than 1%. The figure increases dramatically with older patients or repeated procedures.

Direct and indirect nerve root decompression for herniated discs

Direct methods of nerve root decompression include laminotomy (expansion of the interlaminar space for access to the nerve root and the offending disc fragments), microdiscectomy (laminotomy using a microscope), and laminectomy (total removal of laminae). Methods of indirect nerve root decompression include chemonucleolysis, the injection of chymopapain or other enzymes to dissolve the inner disc. Such chemical treatment methods are less efficacious than standard or microdiscectomy and have rare but serious complications. Any of these methods is preferable to percutaneous discectomy (indirect, mechanical disc removal through a lateral disc puncture).

Management of spinal stenosis

Usually resulting from soft tissue and bony encroachment of the spinal canal and nerve roots, spinal stenosis typically has a gradual onset and begins in older adults. It is characterized by nonspecific limb symptoms, called *neurogenic claudication* or *pseudoclaudication,* that interfere with the duration of comfortable standing and walking. The symptoms are commonly bilateral and rarely associated with strong focal findings on examination Neurogenic claudication, however, can be confused or coexist with *vascular claudication,* in which leg pain also limits walking. The symptoms of vascular insufficiency can be relieved by simply standing still while relief of neurogenic claudication symptoms usually requires the patient to flex the lumbar spine or sit.

The surgical treatment for spinal stenosis is usually complete laminectomy for posterior decompression. Offending soft tissue and osteophytes that encroach upon nerve roots in the central spinal canal and foramen are removed. Fusion may be considered to stabilize a degenerative spondylolisthesis with motion between the slipped vertebra and adjacent vertebrae. Elderly patients with spinal stenosis who tolerate their daily activities usually need no surgery unless they

develop new signs of bowel or bladder dysfunction. Decisions on treatment should take into account the patient's preference, lifestyle, other medical problems, and risks of surgery. Surgery for spinal stenosis is rarely considered in the first three months of symptoms.

Except for cases of trauma-related spinal fracture or dislocation, fusion alone is not usually considered in the first three months following onset of low back symptoms.

FURTHER MANAGEMENT CONSIDERATIONS

Following diagnostic or surgical procedures, the management of most patients becomes focused on improving physical conditioning through an incrementally increased exercise program. The goal of this program is to build activity tolerance and overcome individual limitations due to back symptoms. At this point in treatment, symptom control methods are only an adjunct to making prescribed exercises more tolerable.

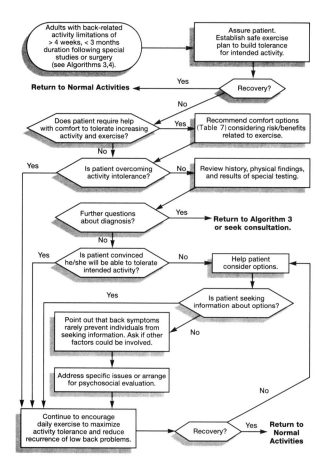

Algorithm 5. Further management of acute low back problem.

- Begin with low-stress aerobic activities to improve general stamina (walking, riding a bicycle, swimming, and eventually jogging).

- Exercises to condition specific trunk muscles can be added a few weeks after. The back muscles may need to be in better condition than before the problem occurred. Otherwise, the back may continue to be painful and easily irritated by even mild activity. Following back surgery, recovery of activity tolerance may be delayed until protective muscles are conditioned well enough to compensate for any remaining structural changes.

- Finally, specific training to perform activities required at home or work can begin. The objective of this program is to increase the patient's tolerance in carrying out actual daily duties.

When patients demonstrate difficulty regaining the ability to tolerate the activities they are required (or would like) to do, the clinician may pose the following diagnostic and treatment questions:

- Could the patient have a serious, undetected medical condition? A careful review of the medical history and physical examination is warranted.

- Are the patient's activity goals realistic? Explor-

ing briefly the patient's expectations, both short- and long-term, of being able to perform specific activities at home, work, or recreation may help the patient assess whether such activity levels are actually achievable.

- If for any reason the achievement of activity goals seems unlikely, what are the patient's remaining options? To answer this question, the patient is often required to gather specific information from family, friends, employers, or others. If, on followup visits, the patient has made no effort to gather such information, the clinician has the opportunity to point out that low back symptoms alone rarely prevent a patient from addressing questions so important to his or her future. This observation can lead to an open, nonjudgmental discussion of common but complicated psychosocial problems or other issues that often can interfere with a patient's recovery from low back problems. The clinician can then help the patient address or arrange further evaluation of any specific problem limiting the patient's progress. This can usually be accomplished as the patient continues, with the clinician's encouragement, to build activity tolerance through safe, simple exercises.

EXCERPTS FROM
BACK PAIN: REPORT OF A CSAG COMMITTEE ON BACK PAIN
by Clinical Standards Advisory Group, HMSO, London, 1994

THE NEED FOR CHANGE IN NHS SERVICES FOR PATIENTS WITH LOW BACK PAIN

The Epidemiology Review (Waddell 1994) shows the scale of the health problem of low back pain and disability. This has not been solved by current clinical management or present NHS [National Health Service] services. We recognize that individual specialists, therapists, and departments do provide a very good service to patients with back pain, incorporating many of the present proposals. Nevertheless, the District Visits show that current clinical standards generally fall short of the ideal suggested in the Management Guidelines. Resources are often devoted to symptomatic treatments which the scientific evidence suggests are either ineffective or sometimes positively harmful (DHSS 1979; Spitzer et al. 1987; Bigos et al. 1994a). Access and availability is subject to long delays, except for emergency and urgent referral for

acute specialty investigation and treatment of serious spinal pathology and acute surgical problems, which is generally satisfactory provided these patients are "fast-tracked." Routine hospital specialty services and referral patterns are largely inappropriate for patients with simple backache. Even when ineffective treatments are not directly harmful they may cause more subtle harm: long delay while awaiting these treatments in itself leads to chronic pain and disability. It also defers the consideration and delivery of more effective management. Overall, there is much ineffective and wasteful use of NHS resources (Waddell 1994).

In 1979 the DHSS Working Group on back pain found "profound and widespread dissatisfaction with what is at present available to help people who suffer from back pain." This situation is unchanged today. All the evidence is that this is unrelated to the reforms resulting from the NHS and Community Care Act

1990. On the contrary, in the District Visits we found that the reforms appeared to be stimulating greater awareness of patients' needs. We found some examples of willingness to consider different and novel ways of providing NHS services to meet these needs. Potentially, the reforms provide the mechanism by which this might be achieved. However, it is important that artificial barriers are not created by the reforms. Purchaser specific contracts for low back pain are recommended to overcome this.

The problems of NHS services for back pain are now widely recognized and, accordingly, we make recommendations on how these services should be reorganized. Our main priority has been to improve standards of care and NHS services to patients with back pain, although these proposals should also lead to more efficient and cost-effective use of resources. Firstly, we consider fundamental principles for such service. We then apply these principles to the provision of support services for the management of simple backache in primary care and to a Back Pain Rehabilitation Service for those patients who do not settle with primary care management.

ACTIVE REHABILITATION

The Epidemiology Review (Waddell 1994) shows that the present problem is not an epidemic of low back pain but rather an epidemic of chronic disability due to simple backache. In the past, backache has generally been managed as a mechanical problem. There is, however, now considerable evidence that back pain and disability are better understood and managed as a clinical syndrome which includes important physical, psychological, and social interactions. Management and advice given to all patients must take full account of the psychosocial and occupational assessment. Some patients will require more specific psychological support and occupational advice.

At present, standard medical management for back pain is by rest and analgesic medication according to orthopedic principles and teaching. There is however no evidence to support the use of rest for simple backache for more than one to three days, and the ill effects of prolonged rest are well recognized. Most treatments used for back pain are symptomatic, and there is little evidence that they have any lasting effect (Koes et al. 1991; Bigos et al. 1994a). Patients do require symptomatic help for pain control, but for a successful final outcome management should also be directed to restoring function by active rehabilitation (Waddell 1993).

An active rehabilitation program should be distinguished from specific back exercises. Individual back exercises may aim to reduce pain, strengthen muscle groups, and improve movement or posture. They are often prescribed as a second stage of management after pain relief and patients are often advised to stop if pain is provoked. An active rehabilitation program uses exercises, but its main emphasis is on restoring full function and regaining physical fitness, and is based on progressively increasing quotas of activity rather than on symptoms of pain. The distinction may be compared with prescribing quadriceps exercises for an elderly patient with a fractured femur or teaching them to walk again.

Most physical therapists do advise, prescribe, or teach various types of back exercises. There is, however, little scientific evidence to support the value of any specific form of back exercise (Koes et al. 1991). There is now scientific evidence supporting active rehabilitation programs as the best means of achieving lasting relief of both pain and disability (Waddell 1993). All physical therapists agree in principle with this latter approach: indeed, these are the fundamental principles of physical therapy and rehabilitation for all other musculoskeletal conditions. One of the main skills and contributions of physical therapy is in rehabilitation and a few NHS departments provide active programs for back pain. However, in practice, few NHS patients with backache actually receive early active rehabilitation. There should be a fundamental change in management strategy directed to early active rehabilitation and return to work. It should be based on assessment of the physical, psychological, and social needs of the individual patient. This requires change in the medical information and advice given to patients. It also requires reorganization of therapy services and a shift of resources to put the principle into practice.

TIME SCALE OF MANAGEMENT

There is clear clinical and epidemiological evidence that the longer the duration of back pain, and particularly work loss, the less successful the outcome of treatment and the lower the chances of getting the patient back to work. The evidence suggests that the first six weeks are crucial in preventing chronicity. By 28 weeks, when Invalidity Benefit commences, there is a high risk of continued chronic pain and disability. Current management and NHS services for back pain are generally outside this time frame. This is a problem common to many NHS services but is of particular relevance to back pain. Long delays while awaiting treatment lead to chronic pain and disability; if the treatment which is then received is ineffective, it would have been better not to have waited for that treatment at all. A fundamental shift in resources is required to provide NHS services to patients with back pain at the acute stage to prevent it becoming chronic.

A BACK PAIN REHABILITATION SERVICE

Better early management and better primary care services should greatly reduce the number of patients with simple backache who need to be referred to hospital. Indeed, ideally, all patients with simple backache would be managed successfully in primary care. We recognize, however, that no matter how much primary care management and services are improved, there will always be some patients with persistent back pain, disability, and failure to return to work. There is a point at which it must be accepted that primary care management has failed and that further measures are required. If the proposals to improve primary care management are implemented and successful, however, the numbers requiring such services should be greatly reduced.

We consider that improved access and availability to secondary care for patients with simple backache can best be achieved by a reorganization of services to meet their specific needs and this was widely supported on the District Visits. This is best described as a Back Pain Rehabilitation Service. It should be a dedicated service because of the numbers involved and the interdisciplinary nature of the resources required, which cut across existing specialty and directorate boundaries. The service should be clearly distinguished in aims, resources, and referral patterns from acute specialty services for the investigation and management of patients with serious spinal pathology or those with nerve root pain who require consideration of surgery.

In principle, the Service could be located wher-

ever the resources can be made available. Ideally, according to the principle of simple backache being managed in primary care, it might best be located in primary care. In terms of getting patients back to work, it might best be located in the workplace as part of an occupational health service. The question might be one for future research and development. However, the multidisciplinary resources required for such a Service are rarely available in either primary care or occupational health services. At present, the staff, resources, logistics, and organization required are most likely to be available and supplied most efficiently from a hospital service.

The Service should be multidisciplinary in nature and approach, although the exact range of specialties and staff might vary with local needs and resources. Ideally, the Service should have the facilities to provide: diagnostic triage and investigation; clinical, psychological, and occupational assessment; pain control facilities; physical therapy including manipulation; an active exercise, functional restoration, and rehabilitation program; counseling; and occupational or vocational rehabilitation. The major emphasis of the Service should be on rehabilitation and the selection of disciplines and staff should be designed to achieve this end. These needs are mainly low-tech, low-cost, and high-volume in nature and should be reflected in the organization, selection of staff, and resources of the service.

The Service should be led by a consultant. Both patients and GPs expect and demand a specialist service. It is also essential for final clinical responsibility and for administrative purposes. Responsibility for the Service should be specified in the consultant's contract, and time allocated in his or her job description. The consultant is most likely to be drawn from orthopedic surgery, rheumatology, rehabilitation medicine, pain management, orthopedic or musculoskeletal medicine, but possibly from primary care, behavioral medicine, or physical therapy. Whatever the main specialty training and contract of the consultant, however, it is important that the consultant's main commitment, responsibility, and job description are to the overall management and rehabilitation of back pain, and not to the provision of individual specialty skills or techniques. The service should be clearly identified and named as a dedicated Back Pain Rehabilitation Service, even if, for administrative purposes, it forms part of an orthopedic surgery, rheumatology, or other directorate.

Many of the resources required for such a Service already exist, and are provided to patients with simple backache. What is needed is more efficient organization of these resources. Medical specialty input should be largely on a sessional basis, e.g., for pain relief techniques. Osteopathic or chiropractic input could also be on a sessional basis. Although the Service should be consultant-led for the reasons given above, much of the service delivery can and should be provided by clinical assistants with a primary care background, by physical therapists or practitioners, and by counseling staff. The Back Pain Rehabilitation Service should work closely with primary care services in the local district and play an important role in continuing education for primary care. Close links will also facilitate efficient referral from and return to continued primary care management. There should be a major emphasis on self-help to prepare patients for their own continued management. Group therapy and support groups are helpful in principle and cost-effective. The Service should liaise with and cooperate with employers and occupational health services to help patients return to work as soon as possible. There may be links and shared resources with an acute pain service and with community physiotherapy services. The main physical resources required are existing outpatient clinics, physiotherapy and occupational therapy accommodation, and relatively low-cost rehabilitation equipment.

Back Pain in the Workplace: Management of Disability in Nonspecific Conditions, edited by W.E. Fordyce, IASP Press, Seattle, © 1995.

8

System Change Proposals

This chapter presents disability management change proposals, the major objective of this report. It addresses what happens after onset of back pain complaints, health care seeking, entry into the health care system, and credible diagnosis as nonspecific low back pain (NSLBP). It assumes that workers will have been assigned temporary disability status after report of a work-related injury. If disability is deemed partial, it assumes the worker will be working part-time and under medical supervision. If deemed total, it assumes the worker is under medical supervision.

Recognizing that NSLBP and disability status considerations relating to it have powerful links to a person's environment makes clear that major changes in disability management policies are essential. Particularly, the purported linkage of NSLBP to anatomical and physiological parameters should be carefully reassessed. The linkage to environmental factors, including but not restricted to psychological factors, themselves so sensitive to environment, should be strengthened. That change is central to the proposals set forth here.

GUIDING PRINCIPLES

1. Management of disability in NSLBP involves a series of interlocking or interdependent systems. These systems include employers or industry, the health care system, compensation payment, medical services and their reimbursement, unemployment programs, individual and family assistance programs, and legal mechanisms for challenging decisions in any of those components. Changes in one component influence one or more of the others, perhaps requiring compensating changes. Changes in these "other" systems, where implied or necessitated, will be noted. Required changes will be assumed to occur.

2. Incentives to health care providers and disability recipients need to be arranged such that they do not promote more enduring disability. This is a particularly important consideration in fee-for-service systems such as in the United States.

3. Medical benefits should be separated from disability benefits. Access to medical benefits should not be determined by or be contingent on formal status as disabled, temporary or permanent, whether or not medical reimbursement is assigned to employer or workers' compensation agency. Insofar as medical services are reimbursed from disability benefit programs for disability-related services, that should occur only within the guidelines set forth below. This in turn means that change will be needed in countries in which medical benefits are organized within the disability management or workers' compensation programs, such as in the United States. Loss of access to medical benefits can be a potent disincentive to ending disability status and return to work.

Remaining on the disability rolls may be the only way the worker can see to provide for health needs. If the worker fails at an attempt to return to work and loses his or her job, dependents may also lose their health care funding. Finally, even if the disabled worker finds new employment, the health insurance offered by the new employer may exclude preexisting conditions. These environmental and economic factors contribute to the disability epidemic and are particularly acute in the United States but are not unknown in other countries. They must be changed as part of the restructuring of the disability system.

OBJECTIVES OF CHANGE

The introductory chapter set forth general objectives of change, which can be restated in summary form:

1. Change should benefit workers, employers, and society in general.

2. Objectives and benefits for workers:

- diminish risks to health resulting from being inappropriately designated as disabled;

- offer high-quality medical care and rehabilitation services;

- target more effectively the problems underlying chronic suffering;

- provide access to opportunities to modify career goals so as to reduce and prevent disability;

- avoid the threats to family integrity from assignment to unwarranted disability status; and

- protect against the threat to disability benefits stemming from soaring medical and disability costs.

3. Objectives and benefits for employers:

- retain and enhance the economic productivity derived from healthy and valued workers; and

- lessen costs for medical services, disability benefits, return-to-work assisting services, and personnel replacement costs for workers lost to disability status.

4. Objectives and benefits for society:

- diminish incidence and duration of disability, with its attendant costs to employers and third-party carriers of medical and disability benefits;

- diminish the risks inherent in excessive medical services;

- reduce the costs of health care by eliminating services not useful for the patient;

- diminish loss of productivity and loss of tax revenues from disabled workers; and

- diminish litigation costs arising from the ambiguities of disability definition and assignment.

IMPLICATIONS OF NSLBP AS ACTIVITY INTOLERANCE

Conceptualizing chronic NSLBP as a "medical" problem implies that medical interventions are required to restore function. Recognizing that the problem is a biopsychosocial phenomenon leads to different strategies for amelioration. The focus should be on restoring activity level. Reliance solely on medically

based interventions to accomplish this must be terminated.

POLICY CHANGE PROPOSALS

Chapter 7 dealt with early management by the health care system of NSLBP as derived from the U.S. Agency for Health Care Policy and Research (AHCPR) Guidelines (Bigos et al. 1994a) and the U.K. Clinical Standards Advisory Group Report (CSAG 1994). Those guidelines address, particularly, pathoanatomical issues pertaining to NSLBP. Chapters 3, 4, and 5 have shown the importance of the interaction between person and environment as a major source of influence on the complaint of pain.

This report and the directions taken by the AHCPR Guidelines and the CSAG Report emphasize that complaints of pain in NSLBP are unlikely to be influenced greatly by existing health care interventions intended to alleviate pain and suffering.

Single-payer health care systems such as the United Kingdom and Canada have proportionally more family physicians relative to specialists. Conversely, the fee-for-service system of the United States has proportionally more specialists relative to family physicians. However, as the data reported in Chapters 2 and 3 indicate, disability rates for NSLBP under both systems have escalated significantly. Under both systems the problem remains and appears to have comparable magnitude. This situation further supports the concept that traditional medical interventions for NSLBP, whether offered by primary care physicians or specialists, have modest relevance.

Information presented in Chapter 6 indicates worksite interventions may have greater effect on subsequent disability rates for NSLBP than does medical treatment. Thus, treatment plans should not be predicated solely on continuing complaints of pain. The assumption that resolution of pain complaints in NSLBP requires modification of some allegedly pertinent body defect can no longer be accepted.

SHIFT TO TIME-CONTINGENT TREATMENT

Subject to a few exceptional circumstances described below, the relationship between complaints of pain and medical interventions should be altered so that treatment is not pain-complaint contingent. Pain complaints in NSLBP are not a reliable index of a continuation of a medical problem, or its magnitude.

The natural course of NSLBP is that return to essentially normal function should be anticipated within six weeks (e.g., Fig. 3, Chapter 2). Without new diagnostic evidence indicating that the problem is not NSLBP, the justification is lacking for continuing to perceive it as an unresolved medical condition.

There is a second reason for a shift from pain-complaint to time-contingent medical care. Pain behavior–contingent disability status can diminish the likelihood the person will return to work irrespective of "medical" considerations. It may promote persistence of disability, similar to a learning or conditioning effect (e.g., Fordyce 1976). The point is illustrated by the history of management of analgesics in chronic pain. Emergence more than 20 years ago of a behavioral science perspective on clinical pain (e.g., Fordyce et al. 1968a, 1968b, 1973) led to a reassessment of methods for scheduling prescribed analgesics for chronic pain. Previously, scheduling analgesics for chronic pain had been on a *prn,* or take only as needed, basis. This arrangement was intended to discourage excessive use and addiction or habituation. Nonetheless, chronic pain patients frequently became physically dependent or habituated to prescribed narcotic analgesics. From a learning or conditioning perspective, *prn* might be expected to promote the conditions, physical dependence and/or habituation, it was designed to minimize (Fordyce 1976; Fordyce et al. 1986). Analgesic delivery thus was shifted away from the adverse conditioning effects of the *prn* strategy, and time-contingent strategy was substituted for a pain behavior–contingent mode. Results quickly demonstrated the validity of the approach (Berntzen and Gotestam 1987; Buckley et al. 1986; Fordyce et al. 1973) and it is now commonplace in health care delivery (Buckley et al. 1986).

This experience with analgesia has potential implications for disability status with sanctioned "time out" from competitive work accompanied by wage replacement funding. Recognition of the potential of pain behavior-contingent consequences for strengthening and maintaining adherence to disability status is important.

In line with the AHCPR Guidelines and the CSAG Report, it is proposed that the duration of support or reimbursement for medical services for NSLBP should be defined by time and not complaint of pain. Correspondingly, the duration of temporary disability status for NSLBP also should be limited. It should be independent of the complaint of pain.

DISABLED VERSUS UNEMPLOYED

Making duration of temporary disability in NSLBP time-contingent influences what happens to wage replacement funding for disability status should the injured worker not resume employment. Resolution of this issue requires attention to incentive/disincentive matters pertaining to return to work, a matter considered in detail in Chapter 9, as well as consideration for support and survival of the worker and his/her family.

One solution to this matter lies in recognizing that activity intolerance is a form of unemployment. We propose that injured workers persisting in activity intolerance beyond the allotted time for medical treatment and temporary disability status be classified as "unemployed." Wage replacement benefits accruing to status as unemployed would continue to apply, as would available return-to-work incentives. This proposal presumes that access to medical services generally, and not just for NSLBP, is part of each society's overall plan and should not be contingent on complaints of work-related NSLBP. Access to medical services contingent upon chronic NSLBP is neither warranted nor provided. This stance is a significant change for societies in which medical services are provided on a fee-for-service basis.

REEVALUATION AS A SAFETY NET

Interpersonal variability is sufficient to warrant provision for exceptional cases falling beyond the time limits proposed and set forth in Fig. 3 (Chapter 2). Injured workers diagnosed as having NSLBP but who fail to return to work within the proposed six-week time interval should undergo comprehensive reevaluation. That reevaluation can serve as the basis for recommending additional time and/or rehabilitation.

THE JOB ACCOUNT CONCEPT

Activity intolerance should not inevitably be seen as a disability for which a medically related intervention might be contemplated. It may be a problem of dissonance between worker characteristics and job characteristics. Such dissonance is commonplace. People often change jobs in response to it. However, a worker does not always have the option of changing to a job providing a "better fit."

Programs need to be devised that enhance opportunity to reduce job-worker dissonance when employer-based job changes are not feasible. Employers often are limited in how much accommodation is possible or economically viable. Expanding worker options for addressing activity intolerance serves to compensate for the reduction of disability as a remedy for difficulties with work. Such a program can benefit employers as well as workers. Under the present impairment-rating system of disability assignment, employers usually are indemnified for worker disabilities, including conditions purporting to be related to or caused by pain resulting from work injury. Programs designed to diminish activity intolerance and resulting in a return to employment reduce employer indemnity. Such programs would also diminish the adverse effects to worker and family of activity intolerance previously misguidedly attributed to work injury and pain. Costs to society from lost productivity could also be offset.

Just as success at a job cannot be guaranteed, so also job happiness or a "good job fit" cannot be guaranteed. Programs to empower the worker to make job changes more easily when problems approaching or reaching activity intolerance occur may be achievable.

The general format might function somewhat like a retirement program and could be tied directly to it. On assuming a new job, an appropriate percentage of wages would go into an individual worker's job account fund. Employers would presumably also contribute to the job account fund. If the worker never draws on the fund, retirement funds would be correspondingly larger. If the worker draws upon the account to explore job changes, to receive further skill or educational training, or to receive some form of remediation designed to enhance job coping or job performance, retirement funds would be correspondingly diminished. The funds would not diminish if the employer instigates these activities. Rates of employer contributions to the fund could be adjusted to promote job longevity. That is, the longer the worker remains in a job, the greater the contribution rate to the fund from the employer.

Rates of contribution for employer and/or for worker might also be adjusted to reflect the probable length of time a worker might reasonably be expected to perform a given kind of work. Jobs requiring greater physical strength or endurance presumably lead to activity intolerance at a more rapid rate. Job funds for such jobs might be programmed to accumulate resources more rapidly to permit earlier shifts to less demanding work.

It is beyond the scope of this report to describe in detail how an individual job account program might be organized. However, the balance between needs of the worker and those of society must be considered in light of a diminished role of disease-model based concepts in disability determination. Job account programs would seem to offer promise of accomplishing this objective.

An important consideration in a job account fund plan is determination of where the initiative lies. Career track choices by workers entering the labor market should be influenced by knowledge about the job account. Decisions as to whether to seek to remain in a particular job or kind of job or to explore alternatives also should be choices of the worker, assuming the employer agrees to retain the worker. This arrangement seems more likely to promote an optimal balance between worker interests and those of employers.

ALGORITHM

An algorithm describing the format for managing low back pain, including both nonspecific (NSLBP) and specific pain, is presented in Fig. 10. The plan provides that failure of workers diagnosed with NSLBP to return to work leads to a comprehensive evaluation involving appropriate medical, psychological, and vocational components. Such evaluation should be made by appropriately experienced profes-

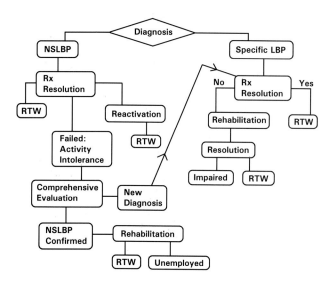

Fig. 10. Algorithm of management of low back pain.

sionals with an understanding of the complex relationship among pain/suffering and personal and emotional functioning and the impact of the social, familial, and work context on patient functioning. All components of the comprehensive evaluation should be integrated into the decision-making process. If that evaluation leads to diagnosis as specific low back pain, the person is referred for appropriate medical management. If, however, the evaluation confirms NSLBP as the appropriate diagnosis, the worker is referred for rehabilitation. If that approach fails to lead to return to work, the worker is reclassified as unemployed.

SUMMARY OF POLICY CHANGE PROPOSALS

Table 9 summarizes these policy change proposals and the approximate time frame for each. Further explanation of the algorithm and Table 9 follows.

- Workers claiming NSLBP are referred for appropriate medical evaluation and, assuming medical evaluation has ruled out specific back pain, placed on temporary disability status.

- Medical benefits accruing to temporary disability status apply automatically for two weeks and contingently for an additional two weeks. The contingencies are that the care-funding agency is provided with a treatment plan directly addressing activity intolerance by reactivation and evidence of established communication with the employer regarding a return-to-work plan. The alternative is credible diagnostic evidence indicating the disabling condition is not NSLBP but a specified pain-related condition qualifying as long-term, per the AHCPR Guidelines (Bigos et al. 1994a) or the CSAG Report (CSAG 1994). Conditions diagnosed as something other than NSLBP would

be withdrawn from further consideration within the framework presented here. In those cases treatment or impairment or disability determination action would derive from policy bearing on the new diagnosis, not on NSLBP.

- Reimbursement for medical services for NSLBP in a fee-for-service system ends with return to work, or with failure to provide and implement a reactivation plan and/or failure to provide evidence of return-to-work communication plans with employer, or with passage of six weeks without return to work. In single payer or contractual medical services systems, authorization for continued treatment should fit the same time standards.

- Worker receives wage replacement funding benefits on a temporary disability basis until return to work, but for no more than six weeks in any case unless credible diagnostic evidence indicates permanent or long-term disability; i.e., diagnosis other than NSLBP.

Failure to return to work

In cases of failure to return to work but without permanent or long-term disability status, the worker is referred to comprehensive, multidisciplinary evaluation, incorporating medical, psychological, and vocational assessment. Options from this assessment are:

- Rediagnosis of medical status as other than NSLBP and referral to appropriate medical facility. This option captures cases in which original diagnosis was inaccurate.

- NSLBP problem correctly diagnosed but judged to have been improperly or inadequately managed, and reactivation and return to work are achievable within two to four weeks. Worker returned to original facility, or to a different facility,

Table 9
Proposed policy, by weeks away from work

	1	2	3	4	5	6	7
Job status	NW	NW	NW	NW	NW	NW	NW
Medical benefits	Y	Y	(Y)	(Y)	(Y)	(Y)	N
Reimbursement for medical services	Y	Y	(Y)	(Y)	(Y)	(Y)	N
Wage replacement benefits	Y	Y	Y	Y	Y	Y	N
Comprehensive rehabilitation					Y	Y	
Classification	D	D	D	D	D	D	UN
Unemployment benefits	N	N	N	N	N	N	Y

Note: NW = not working; Y = yes; (Y) = contingent yes; N = no; D = temporarily disabled; UN = unemployed.

for reactivation and preparation for return to work. Medical reimbursement as in second policy change proposal above; i.e., for two weeks, extendable to four if governing contingencies are met.

- Comprehensive evaluation indicates the core problem is mismatch of worker to job or career track; in which case these options apply:

  - if retraining and/or placement assistance for suitable work is judged to be feasible, referral to vocational planning resource occurs.

  - if retraining and/or placement in suitable work is judged not to be feasible, worker remains on temporary disability until six weeks since onset of disability benefits.

- Comprehensive evaluation indicates psychological problems interfering significantly with reactivation and return to work: referral to appropriate treatment resource. Medical reimbursement derives from a health benefits program as pertains to psychological conditions, not as linked to temporary disability from NSLBP.

If return to work has not occurred at six weeks and a credible reactivation and return-to-work planning program is not underway, the worker is reclassified as unemployed and receives the benefits accorded by the appropriate system or agency. No medical benefits are specific to temporary disability from NSLBP. Medical benefits for any or all conditions, including specific low back pain, are determined by existing medical benefit plans.

Classification as unemployed provides access to such wage replacement funding or family sustenance resources as may exist or be developed in a given society. It also provides access to whatever vocational planning and training resources exist within the programs of the agency mandated to deal with assistance in return to work of the unemployed. Earlier in this chapter we discussed a proposal for provision of resources to assist in changing career track, for vocational training, and in job placement: the job account concept. That proposal is not specific to NSLBP or programs concerned with management of permanent or long-term disability.

EFFECT ON SYSTEM PARTICIPANTS

WORKER AND FAMILY

- Prompt access to diagnostic services and health care for NSLBP geared to restoration of activity

tolerance and return to work and with minimized ambiguity regarding diagnosis and probable course.

- Prompt linkage of medical care with employer to facilitate return to work.

- If return to work does not occur within six weeks, prompt access to comprehensive reevaluation, including psychosocial and vocational appraisal, and prompt referral for such additional services as may be needed.

- If initial diagnosis of NSLBP is changed to another "medical condition," prompt referral for appropriate treatment, restoration of activity level, and facilitation of return to work.

- Wage replacement funding from temporary disability status until return to work or rediagnosis as not NSLBP. Wage replacement funding continues if and as indicated from impairment/disability status of new diagnosis.

- Failure to achieve restored activity level in NSLBP and no return to work leads to reclassification as unemployed.

EMPLOYER

- Integration of medical management with restoration of activity level and return to work.

- Extension of temporary disability indemnity beyond six weeks contingent upon rediagnosis as other than NSLBP.

HEALTH CARE SYSTEM

- Prompt coordination of treatment and reactivation with return to work.

- Timely comprehensive reevaluation if return to work does not occur within six weeks, with appropriate referrals, if indicated.

COMPENSATION AGENCY/INSURANCE CARRIER

- Prompt coordination of medical management with restoration of activity level and return to work.

- Timely reevaluation if return to work not achieved and integration of psychosocial and vocational factors into case management.

- NSLBP classified as temporary disability with time-limited wage replacement funding unless rediagnosis leads to new classification.

SOCIETY

- Integration of health care with return to productivity.

- Integration of disability and unemployment benefits with realistic appraisal of impairment and disability status.

SPECIAL ISSUES IN FEE-FOR-SERVICE SYSTEMS

1. Some physicians, anticipating possible loss of medical benefits for their patients after six weeks, may be too quick to order expensive and perhaps marginally indicated imaging studies. Standards for use of imaging techniques, per the AHCPR Guidelines and the CSAG Report (Chapter 7; Bigos et al. 1994a; CSAG 1994), and cost control forces within managed care systems should diminish or contain this issue.

2. Anticipation of a need or desire to extend treatment authorization in cases diagnosed as NSLBP could encourage use of back pain–related diagnostic labels implying specificity when such may be only speculative during the four- to six-week observation period. Alternatively, time-limited treatment and temporary disability status for NSLBP may encourage greater use of diagnostic labels having psychologic or psychiatric linkage; e.g., one of the somatoform disorders, cumulative trauma disorders.

Chapter 5 discusses relationship of pain to psychologic/psychiatric disability. Resolution of this issue rests ultimately in an analysis of the scope and limits of the use of temporary or permanent disability status for those kinds of diagnostic categories. The position is that they are psychologic/psychiatric issues not having primary roots in back pain

3. Monitoring of physician diagnostic activities must be established to ensure that patients with NSLBP are not assigned to other diagnostic groups that permit the delivery of unneeded health care and the prolongation of sanctioned disability.

LONG-TERM SUFFERING AS A SOCIAL PROBLEM

Placing long-term disability status and attendant benefits for NSLBP on a time-contingent basis reduces excessive and unproductive long-term medical management of NSLBP, diminishes incentives for remaining on disability status for low back pain, and reduces employer expenditures for long-term disability. It is also mindful of the need to provide a "safety net" for workers and families. The plan does not alter the fact that many persons are chronically suffering and are unable to compete effectively. Those persons present a major policy issue for all societies. These proposals inhibit assignment to incorrect and costly disability status for NSLBP. What becomes of those who cannot compete in the workplace? Some may be classified by comprehensive evaluation as having psychologic-based impairments, from which long-term disability benefits may derive and for which medical benefits suitable to the diagnosed condition may apply. The success or failure of those treatments is a matter for demonstration and observation but does not and should not stand as a criterion for the merits of the proposals set forth here.

Some workers are at a point by virtue of age, physical characteristics, or lack of sufficient skills relative to the evolving demands of work, where no viable method of providing a "level playing field" for competitive effort and opportunity exists. It becomes a social policy issue as to whether retirement status with attendant sustenance benefits is an option before reaching the prevailing retirement age for the society involved. The issue can be posed another way. Setting retirement age and associated benefits at an arbitrary figure, such as 65, as is generally true in the United States, assumes everyone "wears out" at the same rate or that retirement benefits are a function of chronology, not "wear out." That issue should be between the worker and his/her family and society; not between worker and employer. The exceptions presumably apply to employment arrangements that include provision for early retirement under suitable conditions and with appropriate retirement benefits. The job account fund proposal suggests a partial remedy to this problem.

LEGAL RECOURSE ISSUES

The fundamental issue of the relationship of the individual to society and its administrative mechanisms underlies these policy change proposals. LaRocca, in an editorial introduction to the Quebec Report (Spitzer et al. 1987) notes, "the legal prerogative of individuals who consider themselves to have been injured, whether justly so or not, will disrupt any foreordained time sequence (pertaining to management of disability status)." The place of legal challenges to system decisions as, for example, formulated here, is a social and legal issue. This report seeks to provide a balanced perspective between the needs and rights of the individual and the needs and rights of society, as an embodiment of the needs and rights of all other individuals. It becomes the task of the legal mechanisms by which individual challenges to social "rules" are expressed to make individual determinations. This report has addressed the consequences of alternative determinations. The effects of unfettered litigation on any attempt to change existing systems are difficult to determine.

UNRESOLVED ECONOMIC ISSUES

Economic policy issues unresolved here include methods of "taxation" and payment for career-track reassessment and assistance and for retirement for the reasons set forth immediately above. In the absence of adequate funding from job account plan strategies, who pays and when? This is a crucial issue and an essential adjunct to these change proposals, which must be addressed and should be on the agenda for study and action for each society involved.

Incentives for return to work must be arranged to find a suitable balance between worker and employer and between unemployment benefits and gainful employment. Incentives to employers for accommodating return-to-work arrangements are also important. Finally, the issue of incentives should be addressed with respect to litigation. At present litigation provides an important "safety net" function for injured workers "mis-treated" by the disability system. That function can serve to inhibit individual effort toward restoration of employment.

Back Pain in the Workplace: Management of Disability in Nonspecific Conditions, edited by W.E. Fordyce, IASP Press, Seattle, © 1995.

9

Management of Long-Term Disability

RESTATEMENT OF PROPOSED CONCEPTUAL CHANGES

This chapter concerns management of long-term disability in workers with nonspecific low back pain (NSLBP). Restating proposed conceptual changes should be helpful.

1. NSLBP is redefined as a problem of activity intolerance, not a "medical" condition.

2. NSLBP is considered as temporary and not permanent disability.

3. Complaints of pain, per se, are not adequate to define a medically based pain problem.

4. Psychological factors identified as critical to a worker's activity intolerance (inability to work) might be diagnosed as a psychological but not a pain disability. That could lead to referral for appropriate remediation. Alternatively, activity intolerance could be categorized as a remediable element of a temporary disability status for NSLBP. In either case, disability status as NSLBP should not continue beyond the limits set forth in Chapter 8 without comprehensive evaluation.

If system changes proposed in this report are applied effectively, thereafter the pool of people with long-term disability from NSLBP would be made up of those who were awarded disability status prior to implementation of the proposed changes or who failed to return to work irrespective of the interventions provided and have become classified as unemployed. Permanent disability from NSLBP as a "medical condition" should no longer be an option. It could become so only where medical management has itself produced a "medical condition," i.e., iatrogenically induced specific back pain. Temporary or permanent disability status for other diagnosed specific back pain conditions remain as options but are not the subject of this report.

OBJECTIVES OF LONG-TERM MANAGEMENT

1. Preserve and optimize worker health.

2. Preserve, so far as is practicable, the health and economic viability of the family unit.

3. Enable long-disabled patients to return to work when possible.

4. Minimize unnecessary health care services.

5. Minimize need for worker to seek medical recertification as disabled.

6. Redirect health care services where indicated by rediagnosis.

7. Reduce litigation.

Whatever the reasons, some people with NSLBP have or will reach long-term disability status. How are they to be helped? First, medical status should be clarified. Clear evidence that the injured worker has an impairment from which permanent or long-term disability status should be derived indicates the problem is not properly labeled as NSLBP, and appropriate referral for remediation should occur. If, however, the problem is NSLBP, a comprehensive evaluation should assess whether anatomical or physiological reasons account for persisting activity intolerance. It should assess whether those limitations have reasonable prospect of being remedied by systematic reactivation and guided reintroduction to competitive employment.

Evaluation should also assess whether psychosocial factors may be influencing worker activity intolerance. Are there psychological problems compromising ability to work or making disability status a better "tradeoff" than working?

Are there effective disincentives to return to work, for example, skill or performance problems on the job, family and social milieu encouragement for continuing deactivation, efforts to enhance access to health care services by maintaining disability status? Is persistence in disability status driven by employer reluctance to reemploy persons with NSLBP or histories of recurring disability episodes? Is it driven by limited job opportunities?

Any one or a mix of the problems just cited dictate the importance of arranging for a comprehensive evaluation of these long-term NSLBP cases. Sophisticated medical, psychosocial, and vocational assessments should be an integral part of evaluation. In most cases, assessment contact with the spouse, significant other, or family unit will be essential.

OUTCOME OPTIONS OF COMPREHENSIVE REEVALUATION

1.   Patient is determined to have a medically limiting condition other than NSLBP, in which case a medically based judgment as to potential treatability and return to work is made. Disability classification should be changed from NSLBP to the impairment diagnosed. Referral for appropriate treatment should be made. That referral should consider the deleterious effects of disability status for protracted periods. If the judgment is that return to work is a sufficiently probable outcome to merit comprehensive treatment, provision for vocational and psychological management should be an integral part of the patient's program. Assessment of the adequacy of such an intervention should include full recognition that disability status lasting more than a few months has almost certainly created formidable obstacles to return to work. If return to work is not judged to be sufficiently probable to warrant the expenditure of resources involved, long-term disability status might be awarded, not for NSLBP but for whatever medically limiting condition has been identified by comprehensive evaluation.

2.   Injured worker condition is reaffirmed as NSLBP. A judgment must then be made as to potential for reactivation and return to work. If probability is sufficient to merit comprehensive treatment, appropriate referral should occur. Provision for vocational and psychological management should be an integral part of the program. Adequacy of such an intervention should be judged with full recognition that disability status for more than a few months creates formidable obstacles to return to work.

If return to work is not judged to be sufficiently probable to warrant the expenditure of resources in-

volved, a basic social and economic decision is at hand. One option is to reassign the worker as unemployed rather than disabled. This has the effect of avoiding excessive medical expenses delivered inappropriately or ineffectually for long-term NSLBP. Depending upon the distribution of legal and economic responsibilities within the jurisdiction involved, indemnification of the employer may be reduced or absolved. Designation as unemployed also may provide an element of further incentive for return to work by helping worker and family to better recognize the nature of the problem.

Designation as unemployed may leave to the injured worker the major burden for rectifying a situation to some extent due to failures of the health care and disability management systems. This issue raises yet again the nature of the implied social contract between the individual and society. How is responsibility "assigned" or shared among worker, health care and disability management programs, and employers? Each society must arrive at a decision. This issue requires rectification of prior system faults, which, as they apply to NSLBP, usually include overmedicalization that has evolved gradually over many decades. The factors contributing to this evolution are many and complex, some only poorly understood. An interesting and penetrating review and discussion of this matter can be found in Shorter (1992). At this point there is no apparent logical basis for determining a priori the allocation of responsibility between the person and the relevant social programs in the individual case.

DISABILITY MANAGEMENT

Disability management (DM) responsibilities are determined partially on the basis of legal indemnification (e.g., employer, insurance company, governmental compensation agency), partially on the basis of expediency. Owens (1993) has a particularly good discussion of this topic.

Who has the resources to implement effective DM? The complexity of medical and disability management has contributed to the problems addressed in this report. Under existing practices, worker, employer, the health care system, and disability management programs have failed. Health care professionals lack sufficient knowledge and sophistication regarding worksite and vocational factors to assume overall disability management responsibility. Conversely, employer-based expertise is clearly insufficient to assume major direction of medical assessment and, where indicated, medical referral or treatment.

The principal functions to be performed by DM are essentially monitoring. In the case of NSLBP, surveillance and monitoring of early health care system management is essential to ensure meaningful plans for reactivation and timely return to work. The expertise that is needed is not worksite procedures to minimize or prevent disability from NSLBP. It is not medical assessment. It is not vocational guidance and assistance in return to work or in modification of career directions. It is a system or network appraisal to ensure the needed components to the overall program are occurring and in a timely and integrated manner.

Employers have an important role in preventing onset of NSLBP and in facilitating return to work. Employers also can make potential contributions to management of long-term disability for NSLBP. Where continuing employer indemnity exists, monitoring by employer-based disability management personnel may be needed to promote assessment of potential for return to work and consideration of job modifications or exploration of alternative types of work. Coordination and integration of vocational and reactivation efforts with opportunities in the worksite clearly should occur.

Allocation of responsibility for DM resides ultimately in legal and economic considerations. DM might occur under the auspices of employers, insurance carriers, or as a governmental function. It might occur as part of comprehensive health care. The choice depends upon social, legal, and economic pol-icy and structures of each society. Whatever the choice, DM should be seen as an essential system monitoring function that transcends the expertise of industry, health care, and vocational professionals. It requires sufficient administrative authority to foster change when a component of the system is functioning in a defective manner.

CONCLUSION

Management of disability for NSLBP is a many-faceted problem. This report has analyzed the dimensions of the problem. Extant knowledge and task force membership expertise have been drawn upon to formulate proposals for change and to provide their rationale. As noted in the first chapter, this report is not a mandate for change; it is a blueprint. It represents the collective effort of many persons.

We conclude that existing disability programs are a major contributor to the explosion in disability ascribed to nonspecific low back pain. We call for a new paradigm for the assessment and management of disability ascribed to low back pain. The new program should have a primary goal of reducing worker pain, suffering, and loss of the economic and personal rewards of gainful employment. We believe that the costs of such a program should accrue to both worker and employer in a fashion that provides appropriate incentives for each to reduce injuries and disability. Major changes are also needed in health care delivery for low back pain. Disability has complex social, personal, and physical antecedents. It is time to change our strategies for its containment.

Bibliography

Abenheim, L. and Suissa, S., Importance and economic burden of occupational back pain: a study of 2500 cases representative of Quebec, J. Occup. Med., 29 (1987) 670.

Adam, G., Interoception and Behavior, Akademiai Kiado, Budapest, 1967

Allan, D.B. and Waddell, G., An historical perspective on low back pain and disability, Acta Orthop. Scand., 234 (Suppl.) (1989) 1–23.

American Psychiatric Association staff, Diagnostic and Statistical Manual of Mental Disorders: DSM-IV, 4th ed., American Psychiatric Association, Washington, D.C., 1994.

Andersson, G., Svensson, H. and Anders, O., The intensity of work recovery in low back pain, Spine, 8 (1983) 880–885.

Battié, M.C., Minimizing the impact of back pain: workplace strategies, Seminars in Spine Surgery, 4, 1 (1992) 20–28.

Battié, M.C., Bigos, S.J., Fisher, L.D., Fordyce, W.E. and Gibbons, L.E., The effect of psychosocial and workplace factors on back-related and other industrial injury claims, Presented at the annual meeting of the International Society for the Study of the Lumbar Spine, Marseilles, France, June 15–19, 1993.

Berkowitz, M. and Berkowitz, E., Rehabilitation in the work injury program, Rehab. Counsel. Bull., 34 (1991) 182–196.

Berntzen, D. and Gotestam, K., Effects of on-demand versus fixed-interval schedules in the treatment of chronic pain with analgesic compounds, J. Consult. Clin. Psych., 55 (1987) 213–217.

Bigos, S. and Battié, M., The impact of spinal disorders in industry. In: J. Frymoyer (Ed.), The Adult Spine: Principles and Practice, Raven Press, New York, 1991, pp. 147–153.

Bigos, S.J., Battié, M.C., Spengler, D.M., Fisher, L.D., Fordyce, W.E., Hansson, T., Nachemson, A.L. and Zeh, J., A longitudinal prospective study of industrial back injury reporting, Clin. Orthop., 279 (1992) 21–34.

Bigos, S. (panel chairperson) et al., Acute Low Back Problems in Adults, Clinical Practice Guideline, AHCPR Publication no. 95-0642, U.S. Department of Health and Human Services, Public Health Service, Agency for Health Care Policy and Research, Rockville, Md., 1994a.

Bigos, S. (panel chairperson) et al., Acute Low Back Problems in Adults: Assessment and Treatment, Quick Reference Guide for Clinicians, AHCPR Publication no. 95-0643, U.S. Department of Health and Human Services, Public Health Service, Agency for Health Care Policy and Research, Rockville, Md., 1994b.

Blow, R.J. and Jayson, M.I.V., Back pain. In: F.C. Edwards, P.I. McCallum and P.J. Taylor (Eds.), Fitness for Work, The Medical Aspects, Vol. 9, Oxford University Press, Oxford, 1988, p. 142.

Bombardier, C., Baldwin, J.L. and Crull, L., The epidemiology of regional musculoskeletal disorders: Canada. In: N.M. Hadler and D.D. Gillings (Eds.), Butterworths International Medical Reviews, Rheumatology and Arthritis in Society: The Impact of Musculoskeletal Diseases, Butterworth, Kent, 1985, pp. 21–29.

Bonica, J.J., Importance of the problem. In: S. Andersson, M. Bond, M. Mehta and M. Swerdlow (Eds.), Chronic Noncancer Pain, MTP Press Limited, Lancaster, UK, 1987, p. 13.

Bonica, J.J., Definitions and taxonomy of pain. In: J.J. Bonica, with J.D Loeser, C.R. Chapman and W.E. Fordyce (Eds.), The Management of Pain, 2nd ed., Vol. 1, Lea and Febiger, Philadelphia, 1990, p. 18.

Bortz, W.M., The disuse syndrome, West. J. Med., 141 (1984) 691–694.

Boschen, K.A., Early intervention in vocational rehabilitation, Rehab. Counsel. Bull., 32 (1992) 254–265.

Brattberg, G., Thorsland, M. and Wikman, A., The prevalence of pain in general population: the results of a postal survey in a county of Sweden, Pain, 37 (1989) 215–222.

Brown, J.A.C., The Social Psychology of Industry, Penguin Books, Baltimore, 1954, pp. 67–68.

Buckley, F.P., Sizemore, W.A. and Charlton, J.E., Medication management in patients with chronic non-malignant pain: a review of the use of a drug withdrawal protocol, Pain, 26 (1986) 153–165.

Budd, M.A., Human suffering: the road to illness or the gateway to learning? Paper presented at Lee Travis Institute for Biopsychosocial Research and the U.S. Public Health Service, Boston, Mass., 1992, pp. 1–17.

Cameron, L., Leventhal, E. and Leventhal, H., Symptom representations and affect as determinants of care seeking in a community-dwelling, adult sample population, Health Psychol. 12 (1993) 171–179.

Cassell, E.J., Recognizing Suffering, Hastings Center Report, May–June 1991, pp. 24–31.

Chelius, J., Galvin, D. and Owens, P., Disability: it's more expensive than you think, Business and Health, 10(4) (1992) 80.

Chöler, U., Larsson, R., Nachemson, A. and Peterson, L.-E., Ont I ryggen: försök med vårdprogram för patienter med lumbala smärttillstånd. Sjukvårdens planerings- och rationaliseringsinstitut, Stockholm, Spri rapport 188, 1985, pp. 1–148.

CSAG (Clinical Standards Advisory Group), Back Pain: Report of a CSAG Committee on Back Pain, HMSO, London, 1994.

Crook, J., Rideout, E. and Browne, G., The prevalence of pain in a general population, Pain, 18 (1984) 299–314.

Cypress, B.K., Characteristics of physician visits for back symptoms: a national perspective, Am. J. Pub. Health, 73 (1983) 389.

Dahlstrom, W.G., Welsh, G.S. and Dahlstrom, L.E., An MMPI Handbook, Vol. I, University of Minnesota Press, Minneapolis, 1972.

Deyo, R. and Tsui-Wu, Y., Descriptive epidemiology of low back pain and its related medical care in the United States, Spine, 12 (1987) 264.

Deyo, R., Diehl, A. and Rosenthal, M., How many days of bed rest for acute low back pain? A randomized clinical trial, N. Engl. J. Med., 315 (1986) 1064–1070.

DHSS, Working Group on Back Pain, HMSO, London, 1979.

Engel, B.T., Nikoomanesh, P. and Schuster, M., Operant conditioning of rectosphincteric responses in the treatment of fecal incontinence, N. Engl. J. Med., 290 (1974) 646–649.

Feuerstein, M., Testimony before the New York Assembly Joint Hearings on Workers' Compensation, University of Rochester Medical Center, Rochester, N.Y., personal communication, 1993.

Fordyce, W.E., Behavioral Methods for Chronic Pain and Illness, C.V. Mosby, St. Louis, 1976, pp. 236.

Fordyce, W., Fowler, R. and DeLateur, B., An application of behavior modification technique to a problem of chronic pain, Behav. Res. Ther., 6 (1968a) 105–107.

Fordyce, W., Fowler, R., Lehmann, J. and DeLateur, B., Some implications of learning in problems of chronic pain, Journal Chronic Disease (1968b) 179–186.

Fordyce, W., Fowler, R., Lehmann, J., Delateur, B.J., Sand, P.L. and Trieschmann, R.B., Operant conditioning in the treatment of chronic clinical pain, Arch. Phys. Med. Rehabil., 54 (1973) 399–408.

Fordyce, W.E., Brockway, J.A., Bergman, J.A. and Spengler, D., Acute back pain: a comparison of behavioral vs. traditional medical management methods, J. Behav. Med., 9 (1986) 127–140.

Fordyce, W., Bigos, S., Battié, M. and Fisher, L, MMPI Scale 3 as a predictor of back injury report: what does it tell us?, Clin. J. Pain, 8 (1992) 222–226.

Frank, A., Regular review: low back pain, BMJ, 306 (1993) 901–909.

Frymoyer, J.W., Back pain and sciatica, N. Engl., J. Med., 318 (1988) 291.

Frymoyer, J. and Cats-Baril, W., An overview of the incidences and costs of low back pain, Orthop. Clin. North Am., 22 (1991) 263–271.

Galvin, D.E., Employer-based disability management and rehabilitation programs, Ann. Rev. Rehabil., 1992, 173–215.

Gyntelberg, F., One year incidence of low back pain among male residents of Copenhagen aged 40–59, Dan. Med. Bull., 21 (1974) 30–36.

Habeck, R., Leahy, M., Hunt, H., Chang, F. and Welch, E., Employer factors related to workers' compensation claims and disability management, Rehab. Counsel. Bull., 34 (1991) 210–226.

Habeck, R.V., Achieving quality and value in service to the workplace, Work Injury Management, 2 (1993) 2–8.

Habeck, R.V., Personal communication, College of Education, Michigan State University, East Lansing, Mich., 1993.

Hadler, N.M., Illness in the workplace: the challenge of musculo-skeletal symptoms, J. Hand. Surg., 10A (1985) 451.

Hadler, N.M., The predicament of backache, J. Occup. Med., 30 (1988) 449.

Hadler, N.M., Knee pain is the malady—not osteoarthritis, Ann. Intern. Med., 116 (1992) 598–599.

Hadler, N.M., Occupational Musculo-Skeletal Disorders, Raven Press, New York, 1993.

Hadler, N.M., The injured worker and the internist, Ann. Intern. Med., 120 (1994) 163–164.

Hager, W.D., Workers Compensation Back Claim Study, National Council on Compensation Insurance, Boca Raton, Fla., 1993, pp. 1–25.

Hettinger, T., Statistics on diseases in the Federal Republic of Germany with particular reference to diseases of the skeletal system, Ergonomics, 28 (1985) 1720.

Horal, J., The clinical appearance of low back disorders in the city of Gothenburg, Sweden: comparisons of incapacitated probands with matched controls, Acta Orthop. Scand., 118 (Suppl.) (1969) 1.

Hunt, A. and Habeck, R., The Michigan Disability Prevention Study, W.E. Upjohn Institute for Employment Research, Kalamazoo, Mich., 1993, pp. 30.

Jarvinen, K.A.J., Can ward rounds be a danger to patients with myocardial infarction? BMJ, 1 (1955) 318–320.

Kaplan, R.M. and Hartwell, S.L., Differential effects of social support and social network on physiological and social outcomes in men and women with Type II diabetes mellitus, Health Psychol., 6 (1987) 387–398.

Kehlet, H. and Dahl, J., Preemptive analgesia: a misnomer and a misinterpreted technique, APS J., 2 (1993) 122–124.

Kelsey, J.L., Epidemiology of Musculoskeletal Disorders, Oxford University Press, Oxford, 1982.

Kerr, P., The high cost of job injury claims, New York Times, Feb. 22, 1993a, p. C-1.

Kerr, P., Insurance plans are health care quandary, New York Times, Apr. 16, 1993b, p. A-1.

Koes, B.W., Bouter, L.M., Beckerman, H., van der Heijden, G.J. and Knipschild, P.G., Physiotherapy exercises and back pain: a blinded review, Br. Med. J., 302 (1991) 1572–1576.

Krämer, J.S., Personal communication [with A.L. Nachemson], Bochum, Germany, 1989.

Kügelgen, B. and Hillemacher, A., Die lumbale Bandscheibenerkrankung in der ärtzlichen Sprechstunde, Springer, Berlin, 1985.

Lee, P., Helewa, A., Smythe, H.A., et al., Epidemiology of musculoskeletal disorders (complaints) and related disability in Canada, J. Rheumatol., 12 (1985) 1169.

Lee, V.L., Transdermal interpretation of the subject matter of behavioral analysis, Am. Psychol., 47 (1992) 1337–1343.

Lemrow, N., Adams, D., Coffey, R., et al., The 50 most frequent diganosis-related groups (DRGs), diagnoses, and procedures: statistics by hospital size and location, DHHS Publication no. (PHS) 90-3465, Hospital Studies Program Research Note 13, Agency for Health Care Policy and Research, Public Health Service, Rockville, Md., September 1990.

Lindstrom, I., Ohlund, C., Eek, C., Wallin, L., Peterson, L.E., Fordyce, W.E. and Nachemson, A.L., The effect of graded activity on patients with subacute low back pain: a randomized prospective clinical study with an operant-conditioning behavioral approach, Phys. Ther., 72 (1992) 279–293.

Loeser, J.D., Perspectives on pain. In: P. Turner (Ed.), Proceedings of First World Congress on Clinical Pharmacology and Therapeutics, Macmillan, London, 1980, pp. 316–326.

Loeser, J.D., Physicians can create disability, Pain Forum (1995) in press.

Mayer, T.G., Gatchel, R.J., Kishino, N. and Mooney, V., Objective assessment of spine function following industrial injury: a prospective study with comparison group and one-year followup, Spine, 10 (1985) 482–493.

Mayer, T., Mooney, V. and Gatchel, R., Contemporary Conservative Care for Painful Spinal Disorders, Lea and Febiger, Philadelphia, 1991, p. 4.

Melzack, R. and Wall, P.D., Pain mechanisms: a new theory, Science, 150 (1965) 971–979.

Mendelson, G., Psychiatric aspects of personal injury claims, C.C. Thomas, Springfield, Ill., 1988.

Merskey, H. and Bogduk, N. (Eds.), Classification of Chronic Pain: Descriptions of Chronic Pain Syndromes and Definitions of Pain Terms, 2nd ed., IASP Press, Seattle, 1994, p. 210.

Nachemson, A.L., Advances in low-back pain, Clin. Orthop., 200 (1985) 266–278.

Nachemson, A.L., Low Back Pain: Causes, Diagnosis and Treatment (in Swedish), Swedish Council of Technology Assessment in Health Care, Stockholm, 1991.

Nachemson, A.L., Newest knowledge of low back pain: a critical look, Clin. Orthop., 279 (1992) 8–20.

Osterweis, M., Kleinman, A. and Mechanic, D., Pain and Disability: Clinical, Behavioral, and Public Policy Perspectives, Institute of Medicine, National Academy Press, Washington, D.C., 1987.

Owens, P., Insurance issures and trends: a focus on disability management, including rehabilitation. In: Private Sector Rehabilitation: Insurance Trends and Issues for the 21st Century. Switzer Monograph (unpublished). National Rehabilitation Association, Alexandria, Va., 1993.

Pennebaker, J.W., The Psychology of Physical Symptoms, Springer Verlag, New York, 1982.

Philips, H.C. and Grant, I., The evolution of chronic back pain problems: a longitudinal study, Behav. Res. Ther., 29 (1991) 435–441.

Powers, W.T., Feedback: beyond behaviorism, Science, 179 (1973) 351–356.

Price, D.D., The question of how the dorsal horn encodes sensory information. In: T.H. Yaksh (Ed.), Spinal Afferent Processing, Plenum, New York, 1986, pp. 445–468.

Raspe, H., Back pain. In: A.J. Silman and M.C. Hochberg (Eds.) Epidemiology of the Rheumatic Diseases, Oxford University Press, Oxford, 1993.

Redd, W.H., Stimulus control and extinction of psychosomatic symptoms in cancer patients in protective isolation, J. Consult. Clin. Psychol., 48 (1980) 448–455.

Riksförsäkringsverket, Den ersatta sjukfranvarons diagnoser, Statistisk rapport, Riksjörskäkrrugs Verbets Rapporter IS-R 5 (1973) 1.

Robertson, L. and Keeve, J., Worker injuries: the effects of workers compensation and OSHA inspections, J. Health Polit. Policy Law, 8 (1983) 581–597.

Roessler, R.T., A conceptual basis for return to work interventions, Rehab. Counsel. Bull., 32 (1988) 205–214.

Romano, J., Turner, J., Friedman, L., Bulcroff, R., Jensen, M., Hops, H. and Wright, S., Observational assessment of chronic pain patient–spouse behavioral interactions, Behav. Res. Ther., 22 (1991) 549–567.

Rousmaniere, P., Stop workers comp from shooting holes in corporate profits, Corporate Cashflow (1990).

Shorter, E., From Paralysis to Fatigue: A History of Psychosomatic Illness in the Modern Era, Free Press, New York, 1992, 419 pp.

Snook, S.H., The costs of back pain in industry, Spine: State of the Art Reviews, 2 (1987) 1.

Snook, S. and Webster, B., The cost of disability, Clin. Orthop., 221 (1987) 27.

Social Security Statistical Supplement, 1977–1979, p. 129, Table 197, 1979.

Spangfort, E., The low back pain problem. In: R. Dubner, G.F. Gebhart and M.R. Bond (Eds.), Proceedings of the Vth World Congress on Pain, Pain Research and Clinical Management, Vol. 3, Elsevier, Amsterdam, 1988, pp. 238–243.

Spengler, D., Bigos, S., Martin, N.A., Zeh, J., Fisher, L. and Nachemson, A., Back injuries in industry: a retrospective study. I. Overview and cost analysis, Spine, 11 (1986) 241–245.

Spitzer, W., LeBlanc, F., et al., Scientific approach to the assessment and management of activity-related spinal disorders, Report of the Quebec Task Force on Spinal Disorders, Spine, 12:7S (European ed., Suppl. 1) (1987) S1–S59.

Sternbach, R.A., Survey of pain in the United States: the Nuprin Pain Report, Clin. J. Pain, 2 (1986) 49–53.

Taylor, H.K. and Curran, N.M., The Nuprin Pain Report, Louis Harris and Associates, New York, 1985.

Troup, J.P., Foreman, T.K., Baxter, C.E. and Brown, D., The perception of back pain and the role of psychophysical tests of lifting capacity, 1987 Volvo Award in Clinical Sciences, Spine, 12 (1987) 645–657.

United States Department of Commerce, Statistical Abstracts, 113th ed., Tables 579 and 587, 1993.

Valkenburg, H.A. and Haanen, H.C.M., The epidemiology of low back pain. In: A.A. White III and S.L. Gordon (Eds.), Symposium on Idiopathic Low Back Pain, C.V. Mosby, St. Louis, 1982, pp. 9–22.

Volinn, E., Theories of back pain and health care utilization, Neurosurg. Clin. N. Am., 2 (1991) 739–748.

Volinn, E., VanKoevering, D. and Loeser, J., Back sprain in industry: the role of socioeconomic factors in chronicity, Spine, 16 (1991) 542–548.

Von Korff, M. and Dworkin, S., An epidemiologic comparison of pain complaints, Pain, 32 (1989) 173–183.

Von Korff, M., Dworkin, S.F. and LeResche, L., Graded chronic pain status: an epidemiologic evaluation, Pain, 40 (1990) 279–291.

Waddell, G., A new clinical model for the treatment of low back pain, Spine, 12 (1987) 632–644.

Waddell, G., Biopsychosocial analysis of low back pain, Baillières Clin. Rheumatol., 6 (1992) 523–557.

Waddell, G., Simple low back pain: rest or active exercise? Ann. Rheum. Dis., 52 (1993) 317–319.

Waddell, G., The epidemiology of back pain. In: Clinical Standards Advisory Group, Epidemiology Review: The Epidemiology and Cost of Back Pain, Annex to the Clinical Standards Advisory Group's Report on Back Pain, HMSO, London, 1994, pp. 1–64.

Waddell, G., Newton, M., Henderson, I., Sommerville, D. and Main, C., A fear-avoidance beliefs questionnaire (FABQ) and the role of fear-avoidance in chronic low back pain and disability, Pain, 52 (1993) 157–168.

Wall, P.D., The John J. Bonica Distinguished Lecture: Stability and instability of central pain mechanisms. In: R. Dubner, G.F. Gebhart and M.R. Bond (Eds.), Proceedings of the Vth World Congress on Pain, Pain Research and Clinical Management, Vol. 3, Elsevier, Amsterdam, 1988, 13–24.

Walsh, K., Cruddas, M. and Coggon, D., Low back pain in eight areas of Britain, J. Epidemiol. Community Health, 46 (1992) 227–230.

Wiesmann, J. and Deyo, R., Back pain: epidemiologic data, APS Bulletin, 3, 1 (1993) 14, 23.

Wood, P.H.N. and Bradley, E.M., Epidemiology of back pain. In: M.I.V. Jayson III (Ed.), The Lumbar Spine and Back Pain, Churchill Livingstone, London, 1987, pp. 1–15.

World Health Organization, International Classification of Impairments, Disabilities, and Handicaps, World Health Organization, Geneva, 1980.

Yaksh, T.L. and Abram, S.E., Preemptive analgesia: a popular misnomer, but a clinically relevant truth? APS J., 2 (1993) 116–121.

Yelin, E., The myth of malingering: why individuals withdraw from work in the presence of illness, Milbank Quarterly 64:4 (1986) 622–648.

Yelin, E., Disability policy: restoring socioeconomic independence, Milbank Quarterly 67 (Suppl. 2, Part 1) (1989).

Yelin, E., Nevitt, M. and Epstein, W., Toward an epidemiology of work disability, Milbank Memorial Fund Quarterly/Health and Society 58:3, Milbank Memorial Fund and Massachusetts Institute of Technology, 1980.

Zola, I.K., Pathways to the doctor—from person to patient, Soc. Sci. Med., 7 (1973) 677–689.

Zuidema, H., National statistics in The Netherlands, Ergonomics, 28 (1985) 3.

Index